The Whole30 Slow Cooker

Cookbook

100 Easy and Delicious Recipes for Rapid Weight Loss. Lose Up to 20 Pounds in 21 Days

Carmela Madison

© Copyright 2020 Carmela Madison All Right Reserved.

In no way it is legal to reproduce, duplicate, or transmit any part of this document by other electronic means or printed format. Any recording of this publication is strictly prohibited, and any storage of this material is not allowed unless with a written permission from the publisher. All rights reserved.

The information provided herein is stated to be truthful and consistent, in that any liability, regarding inattention or otherwise, by any use or abuse of any policies, processes, or directions contained within is the solitary and complete responsibility of the recipient reader. Under no circumstances will any legal liability or blame be held against the publisher for any reparation, damages, or monetary loss due to the information herein, either directly or indirectly.

Legal Notice:

This book is copyright protected. This is only for personal use. You cannot amend, distribute, sell, use, quote or paraphrase any part or the content within this book without the consent of the author or copyright owner. Legal action will be pursued if it is breached.

Disclaimer notice:

Please note the information contained within this document is for educational and enchainment purposes only. Every attempt has been made to provide accurate, up to date, complete and reliable information. No warranties of any kind are expressed or implied. Readers acknowledge that the author is not engaged in the rendering of legal, financial, medical or professional advice.

By reading this document, the reader agrees that under no circumstances are we responsible for any losses, direct or indirect, which are incurred as a result of the use of information contained in this document, including but not limited to errors, omissions, or any inaccuracies

Contents

Introduction 9

Understanding the Whole30 Diet 11

What is a Whole30 diet and what are its basics? 11

Advantages and benefits of the Whole30 diet 12

Possible Cons of the Whole30 Diet 14

What to eat on a Whole30 diet 16

Foods to Avoid on a Whole30 diet 18

Keys of a successful Whole30 diet 19

What is a slow cooker? 20

Advantages of using a Slow Cooker 21

Slow Cooker Times and temperatures 23

Slow cooker tips 25

Slow cooker Safeguards 26

CHAPTER 2: WHOLE30 SLOW COOKER RECIPES 29

Whole30 Slow Cooker Lamb Recipes 31

Recipe 1: Rack of lamb with thyme and rosemary 31

Recipe 2: Slow cooked Rolled lamb 32

Recipe 3: Moroccan style lamb stew 33

Recipe 4: Slow cooked Rolled lamb 34

Recipe 5: Lamb casserole with spinach and kale 35

Recipe 6: Slow cooked Lamb meatballs 36

Recipe 7: Lamb Curry 38

Recipe 8: Spicy Lamb kheema with peas 39

Recipe 9: Slow cooked lamb with sweet potatoes 40

Recipe 10: Lamb Tagine with olives 41

Whole30 Slow Cooker Pork Recipes 43

Recipe 11: Spicy pulled pork 45

Recipe 12: Pork with orange juice 46

Recipe 13: Ham Chowder 47

Recipe 14: Cajun pork 48

Recipe 15: Pork Chili 49

Recipe 16: Slow cooked pork chops with chipotle 50

Recipe 17: Pork Carnitas 51

Recipe 18: Cuban-style pulled pork 52

Recipe 19: Pork with orange juice 53

Recipe 20: Pork patties 55

Whole30 Slow Cooker Beef Recipes 57

Recipe 21: Beef with broccoli 58

Recipe 22: Slow cooked ground beef casserole with cabbage 59

Recipe 23: Slow cooked ground beef casserole with cabbage 60

Recipe 24: Spicy Beef Chilli 61

Recipe 25: Barbecue beef with cabbage Coleslaw 62

Recipe 26: Beef stew 64

Recipe 27: Beef with mango 65

Recipe 28: Shepherd's Pie 66

Recipe 29: Beef Picadillo 67

Recipe 30: Slow cooked short beef ribs 68

Whole30 Slow Cooker Seafood Recipes 71

Recipe 31: Fish Curry with coconut milk 72

Recipe 32: Spicy Garlicky Octopus 73

Recipe 33: Spicy Salmon with dill 74

Recipe 34: Slow cooked Seafood gumbo 75

Recipe 35: Shrimp Scampi 76

Recipe 36: Salmon chilli 77

Recipe 37: Shrimp zoodles 78

Recipe 38: Fish cakes with avocado salsa 79

Recipe 39: Slow cooked calamari with olives 81

Recipe 40: Slow cooked Salmon with orange 82

Whole30 Slow Cooker Poultry Recipes 85

Recipe 41: Slow cooked chicken livers with mushrooms 87

Recipe 42: Chicken Fajitas 88

Recipe 43: Artichoke Chicken casserole 89

Recipe 44: Chicken skewers 90

Recipe 45: Chicken with pineapple 91

Recipe 46: Slow cooked Cornish hens with sweet potatoes and green beans 92

Recipe 47: Garlicky chicken drumsticks 93

Recipe 48: Chicken teriyaki 94

Recipe 49: Chicken with Garlic and Citrus 95

Recipe 50: Chicken patties 97

Whole30 Slow Cooker Soup and stew Recipes 99

Recipe 51: Beef and cabbage stew 100

Recipe 52: Sweet potato soup 101

Recipe 53: Liver stew 102

Recipe 54: Chicken and mushroom soup 103

Recipe 55: Cauliflower soup 104

Whole30 Slow cooker appetizer and snack Recipes 105

Recipe 57: Zucchini rolls 107

Recipe 58: Artichoke and cashews dip 108

Recipe 59: Mashed sweet potatoes 109

Recipe 60: Liver pate 110

Whole30 Slow Cooker Salad Recipes 113

Recipe 61: Beef salad 114

Recipe 62: Sweet potato Salad 115

Recipe 63: Turkey salad 116

Recipe 64: Lamb salad 117

Recipe 65: Cauliflower salad 118

Recipe 66: Chicken Salad 119

Recipe 67: Chicken Cranberry Salad 120

Recipe 68: Shrimp Salad 121

Recipe 69: Pork salad 122

Recipe 70: Liver salad with hazelnuts 123

Whole30 Slow Cooker dessert Recipes 125

Recipe 71: Apple and cranberry sauce 126

Recipe 72: Chocolate fondue 127

Recipe 73: Sugar-free chocolate fudges 128

Recipe 74: Stuffed apples 129

Recipe 75: Chocolate clusters 130

Recipe 76: Slow cooked peaches 131

Recipe 77: Slow cooked pears with pomegranate 132

Recipe 78: Apple sweet potato mash 133

Recipe 79: Slow cooked apple dessert 134

Recipe 80: Almond granola 135

CONCLUSION 137

Introduction

Let me start this book by expressing my utmost gratitude and appreciation to you for purchasing it and for granting me the opportunity to share with you this dietary journey. When I decided to write this book, my core objective was to make this book readable by all readers of all ages and of all cook stages. I tried my best to help clarify everything about the concept of the Whole30 diet and that of slow cooker. And in doing so, I made sure to keep everything as simple and as easy as possible to understand.

The entire book has been organized by being divided into certain sections. Each section of the book focuses on one topic. To begin with, the book starts by explaining the main basics of the Whole30 diet program, its advantages, the basics of using a slow cooker and you will also be able to explore a wide range of 80 succulent Whole30 recipes that. So what it this entire Whole .30 diet about?

Well, to start with, let me tell you that diets have always interested for one reason, I didn't want to lose my shape and you can say; I was quite obsessed with my health and my body. My love for my body stems from my love for my mother who inspired me and who tried different sorts of diets. So, I have been eating healthy since I was a teenager, when my mother went vegetarian, I followed her steps and gave up on eating meat; then when she adopted a Vegan diet, I followed her as well. And it wasn't until a few years ago that I realized that none of the diets I followed was the right for me. It was okay for me to go Vegetarian, but to be Vegan exhausted me; I started feeling tired all the time, I started losing my appetite; but still not losing weight. And the breaking point was when I couldn't work out the way I used to before; I knew something was wrong. And when I consulted a nutritionist, I figured out that it was all because of my diet.

I suffered from various symptoms and the nutritionist recommended that I start eating some proteins; and I, also, figured out that I used some inconvenient ingredients like sugar, some additives and even flours. I didn't know that my favourite ingredients were toxic to me. A variety of reasons led me to realize that I made a huge mistake by adopting the Vegetarian and Vegan diets. I decided to make a research until I stumbled into what is called the Whole30 diet and looked into that program and I have read about how people were extremely satisfied with this diet and some other people even raved about how much weight they lost in a short period of time.

I learned that there are some basic rules I had to adapt to when adopting the Whole30 diet and compared to the Vegan diet, it hasn't been very difficult. The main point behind the Whole diet is to flush our body and boost energy into our organs during 30 days and there was a condition I had to abide by, it is restricted to weight ourselves during the 30 days of the Whole30 diet. After reading this book, you will find out how much the Whole30 diet will change the way we look, the way we eat and our entire lifestyle.

So, aren't you excited to break out through this Whole30 diet slow cooker cookbook and try a wide variety of delicious dishes that will let you enjoy healthy food you never tasted before as soon as you step into your house after an exhausting day at work? And not only you can enjoy the recipes in this book, but you can share it with your family too, because the recipes you will find are suitable for all people and all tastes.

But before using this whole30 slow cooker cook book; make sure to purchase a programmable slow cooker. I hope you enjoy this cookbook and I hope you will have the best cooking experience ever. Have a nice Whole30 slow cooker recipe trip!

Understanding the Whole30 Diet

What is a Whole30 diet and what are its basics?

Have you ever heard of a diet known as Whole30 diet and have you ever wondered if it is the right diet for you or not? Cheers, you are not the only one who wondered about this revolutionary diet. Many people are searching for the Whole30 diet online and there are many talks about the role this diet plays in considerable weight loss. And many people are praising this diet for the role it plays in improving sleep in addition to a variety of physical as well as psychological health benefits. So what does Whole30 diet mean? What are the advantages and disadvantages of adopting a Whole30 diet?

The Whole30 diet was first developed by Melissa Hartwig and Dallas Hartwig in 2009. It is a diet that is based on a 30-day plan and it has been designed as a resetting program for your foods. In fact, the Whole30 diet, as its name suggests, aims towards helping you change all your eating habits at once and improve your health during a month.

Adopting a Whole30 diet means to cut with many foods and this means you have to give up on some of your favourite, but unfortunately, unhealthy ingredients like dairy products, legumes, grains, soy, sweeteners and sugars. The Whole30 diet cookbook offers you a wider range of healthy alternatives to your favourite recipes. And it may be surprising to you, but this diet offers you a great food freedom, so there are no excuses for you not to try it. Quitting eating sugar can be compared to quitting drugs, it is hard at the beginning, but it will be easier with time.

Well, the Whole30 program is an elimination diet that focuses on restoring your health and changes your approach to meals. This program is based on 80 sumptuous recipes that will help you maintain nutritious as well as balanced daily meals.

The Whole30 dietary program can also be described as a revolutionized version of the diet that approaches food differently. It is indispensable in health, weight, shape and to allergies. For instance, fighting allergies and alleviating its symptoms make a great surprise for people who want to get rid of certain annoying allergies.

In a few words, the Whole30 diet program is a restrictive elimination diet that is based on removing all types of inflammatory drinks and foods that can endanger your health and threaten your life. In your newly-adopted diet, you are only supposed to eat clean food and only use the ingredients allowed on the Whole30 diet. This diet will allow you to start your eating habits from scratch and you will start experiencing the improvements very soon. But keep in mind that it is important that you have to stick this diet for 30 days, not less, and don't try to weigh yourself in these thirty days.

So, briefly, the whole30 diet is very simple; it will change the way you cook, the way you eat the way you look and even the way you think about your food. And after 30 days of adopting this new diet, you will figure out that you want to adopt this diet for the rest of your life.

Advantages and benefits of the Whole30 diet

The Whole30 diet has proven it has a wide range of advantages and benefits, which encouraged more people to start adopting this diet and here are some of the major pros of this diet:

1. The whole30 diet imbibes awareness within you

The Whole30 diet encourages you to choose healthier foods and that starts from the simple activity of shopping. Consequently, this diet encourages you to read the labels the ingredients you purchase before consuming it.

2. The whole30 dietary program is an International program that can be used everywhere

Being a restrictive diet doesn't mean that the Whole30 diet is restricted to be used and adopted by a specific country and specific people. In contrast, this revolutionary diet is easy-to follow in the United States of America, in Australia, in England and wherever you go. And this dietary program allows the consumption of seafood, meat, vegetables, eggs, oil, nut and some limited sorts of fruits which perfectly fits the dietary program of Americans.

3. **The whole30 diet helps boost your body with energy,** reduces feelings of hunger and improves your physical activities. Besides, this diet promises to change your mood and even entire lifestyle.

4. **The whole30 diet is praised for the role it plays in improving your social and inner relationships.** Adopting this diet will help you feel happy and satisfied about your body.

5. **The whole30 diet needs only thirty days of your life to feel happier and look healthier.** This diet may be restrictive to some extent, but it is not as hard as you think it is. You won't lose anything if you try the Whole30 diet for thirty days, if it works, you would have found the diet that you can adopt for ages.

6. **Following a whole30 diet will make you stronger physically and emotionally,** you will be able to learn how to cook for yourself and how to be self-reliant too. This diet will teach that you are okay sometimes, to say no to a cake packed with sugars.

7. **Adopting the whole30 diet won't deprive you from enjoying picnics, your family and friends.**

Going to picnics does not necessarily mean that you have to eat everything you take with you. In order to control your hunger, you can drink water instead of eating food.

8. **If you have chosen the whole30 diet, then you can do it**

Having the willingness to do something can help you achieve it in a shorter time than you imagine. If you want to lose weight, don't wait anymore, because the whole30 diet offer you the opportunity to be healthy and fit like you have always wanted to be.

> **Note**

Despite the fact that the whole30 diet has too many benefits, this does not mean that it is a flawless diet. Each diet has its advantages and its disadvantages. So make sure to keep reading in order to know what the possible risks of adopting this diet so that you can avoid it are.

Possible Cons of the Whole30 Diet

In addition to having a large number of benefits, like any diet, the whole30 diet has some possible risks and cons. For instance, the whole30 diet has some downsides that we shall take into consideration before adopting this diet:

1. The whoel30 diet eliminates most of the dairy products, legumes and grains, yet these two ingredients make two of the most recommended five ingredients of the US Agricultural Department. Indeed, on a whole30 diet, you need to give up on rye, wheat, oat, barley, rice, corn, bulgur, millet, buckwheat, and amaranth as well as all-gluten free alternatives too.

2. **Unless you have a certain food intolerance or allergy, it is compulsory to adopt a whole30 diet.** In fact, many nutritionists recommend eating certain dairy products like milk, eggs and yogurt. Dairy products make an excellent source of potassium, calcium and protein. Besides, dairy products are known for its role in building up the bones and reduce the diabetes and cardiovascular diseases. You can use unsweetened dairy products instead of sweetened ingredients.

3. **Depriving your body of whole grains can reduce the consumption of Vitamin E**, fiber, magnesium, Vitamin B and iron. Moreover, consuming whole grains can help reduce the risk of diabetes, cancer, heart disease and lowering high blood pressure. And many legumes like chickpeas, beans, peanuts, soy foods and lentils can boost a variety of our body functions in comparison to junk and fast food.

4. **Adopting the Whole30 diet removes added all sources of sugar** even natural sweeteners like nectar, agave, maple syrup, coconut sugar and honey and this can badly affect the body. But nutritionists allow a limited amount estimated by 10% of calories per day. Fruit juice is also allowed as a sweetener.

5. The Whole30 restrictions

Because the whole30 diet is too restrictive, some people may end up giving up on this diet too soon before feeling the positive effects of this diet.

> **Note:**

The Whole30 diet has many benefits, but it has some constraints too. Hence, it is better to focus on the foods that offer you all the nutrients your body needs. You need lots of vegetables, healthy fats, whole grains and you need.

What to eat on a Whole30 diet

When it comes to the whole30 diet, it is recommended to know what to eat and what not to eat before heading to the kitchen to cook your foods. And here are the Foods that are allowed on the Whole30 diet:

Poultry and meat:

- Veal
- Pork
- Beef
- Chicken
- Lamb
- Duck
- Turkey

Seafood ingredients:

- Anchovies
- Fish
- Calamari
- Shrimp
- Crab
- Scallops
- Lobster

Dairy Products:

- All types of eggs and all types of mayonnaise made of eggs

Fruits:

- Dried and fresh fruits are both allowed

Vegetables

- All types of vegetables are allowed on whole30 diet

Seeds and Nuts:

- All kinds of Nuts and seeds are allowed
- Nut milks
- Nut flours

Oils and fats:

Healthy vegetable oils include:

- Coconut oil
- Clarified Ghee
- Duck fats
- Clarified butter
- Coffee is allowed on whole30 diet
- Red and green onion
- Green, red and orange bell peppers
- Leek
- Tomatoes
- Kale, spinach and greens
- Potatoes
- Garlic
- Sweet potatoes
- Cilantro
- Mushrooms

- Basil
- Lemons
- Jalapenos
- Limes
- Lemon
- Cucumbers
- Avocados
- Salad greens
- Green leaf lettuce
- romaine lettuce
- Watermelon radishes
- Radishes
- Scallions
- Carrots
- Cabbage
- Celery
- Cauliflower
- Fresh ginger
- Eggplants
- Pasteurized eggs for Cesar dressing and mayonnaise
- Apple
- Compliant sausage

- coconut aminos
- Sesame seeds
- Red pepper flakes
- High quality coffee
- Green tea
- Coconut milk
- Almond butter
- Cocoa powder
- Cinnamon
- Unsweetened Coconut chips
- Oranges
- Bananas
- Grapefruit
- Berries
- Cherries
- Dates
- Unsalted cashews

Frozen Foods:

- Frozen green beans
- Black olives
- Almonds almonds
- Soy free tuna
- White wine vinegar
- Red wine vinegar
- Apple cider vinegar
- Rice vinegar
- Sweet Paprika

Foods to Avoid on a Whole30 diet

During your Whole30-day diet, there are certain foods you need to eliminate from your foods and these foods include the following ingredients:

All types of natural and artificial Sugar and sweeteners:

- Honey
- Raw sugar
- Agave syrup
- Maple syrup

Grains:

All types of grains are not allowed including:

- Corn
- Wheat
- Rice
- Oat

Alcohol:

All sorts of alcohol are not allowed including:

- Wines
- Beer
- Spirits
- Liqueur

Legumes and Pulses:

- Lentils
- Beans

- Peanut butter

Dairy products:

- Goat, cow and even sheep's milk
- Cheese
- Yogurt
- Ice cream
- Pasteurized eggs

Soy:

All soy ingredients are not allowed including:

- Tempeh
- Tofu
- Edamame
- Miso
- Soy sauce

All kinds of additives:

- MSG
- Sulfites
- Carrageenan
- Pizzas are not allowed even cauliflower pizza is not allowed

Keys of a successful Whole30 diet

Adopting The Whole30 diet is a life changing experience that needs some rules to be fruitful and successful. And here some of the major keys of a successful Whole30 diet:

1. During the whole30 diet, you are not allowed to weigh yourself for thirty days.

2. Smoking is prohibited on a whole30 diet, at least thirty days and it is recommended to stop smoking three days before starting your diet.
3. Eat small portions of seafood, eggs and meat; but eat a lot of fruits, natural fats, spices, herbs, seasonings and vegetables.

4. Make sure to use a few ingredients in every meal.

5. Do never consume natural, artificial or added sugar on a Whole30diet.

6. Try to stay away from any form of alcohol and don't even use it while cooking.

7. Do not eat any type of grains like corn, millet, bulgur, rice, etc.

8. Avoid all kinds of legumes, including all types of beans, peas, lentils, peanuts and chickpeas.

9. Do not eat any dairy products, even goat, cow or sheep milk.

10. Do not consume fast food, junk foods, baked goods or any sweets and treats.

11. Stay away from pancakes even pancakes made of gluten free flours.

12. No waffles, tortillas, bread, biscuits, no pizza, no crust, no cereals or brownies.

13. Chips, including tortilla, potato and plantain are not allowed.

> **Note:**

One of the more tangible benefits of the Whole30 diet is that it can help eliminate all toxic elements in your body. Thus, following the whole30diet for 30 days can heal your digestive system; fight any inflammation in your body and can improve the quality of your life as a whole.

Overall, adopting a whole30 diet is a physical and mindful experience that can teach you the healthiest way to eat. You don't need to deprive yourself from all staple foods you love, but you can adjust meals according to the list of foods the whole30 diet allows.

What is a slow cooker?

Did you know that slow cooking is one of the best cooking methods to prepare food as it ensures a rich flavour and tenderness? So what is a slow cooker and how does it work? Indeed, today, what we used to know as Crock-pot has gained great popularity with sales that outpaced all expectations.

The history of the original Crock-Pot dates back to the year 1938, when Irving Naxon, was trying his grandmother's favourite Cholent Stew. Cholent meant a meal that was cooked every Saturday or what was known as Sabbath. Naxon's invention was made of a ceramic pot that and he used electric oil to heat it.

And as the invention came to life, Naxon became the head of the Naxon's Utilities Corp, which was the first to sell the crock pot or what was also known as the Beanery cooker. But the company didn't last for too long and was later bought by Hack Miller's Rival Co Manufacturing in 1970; and it was this company that reintroduced the Beanery cooker as a crock pot. And ever since the reintroduction of the beanery under the new name Crockpot, people loved the new appliance more and started purchasing it more and more.

Using a crock pot was the best way to cook cheaper meat portions to make it tender by cooking it for a long period of time that can last for 8 hours or more. Crock-Pot has become now known as a brand manufactured by the Sunbeam products Inc. The crock pot, which was later known as a slow cooker, has proven itself to be one of the best ways of cooking food.

Slow cookers knew an unrivalled increase in sales with about 4.5 million of slow cookers that were sold last year compared to about 3.2 millions in the year 2005 and according to some reports, it was said that About 4.4 million Crock-Pots were sold last year, compared with 3.2 million in 2005. Jarden slow cooker brand controls more than the third of the market in comparison to its competitors lie West Bend and Hamilton Beach.

The new cooking appliance slow cooker is simple and easy-to use; it is also versatile and you can use it to cook stews, soups, roasts, casseroles and even desserts. Slow cooking has proven its efficacy by its economical aspect; besides it uses little power.

The function of the slow cooker is very simple; in fact, when the food is cooked by using the retained heat in the slow cooker insert. A slow cooker is perfect for cooking tough meat portions. And what is more pleasantly surprising about slow cooker is that it doesn't need you keep checking up on the cooking process; all you have to do is to set your slow cooker; then it will be automatically turned off when the timer beeps.

Advantages of using a Slow Cooker

Slow cookers were created at first in just one style, but today, this cooking appliance is found in different sizes and shapes everywhere in the entire world. There are different types of slow cookers like programmable cookers and manual slow cookers. Today's slow cookers can be square or round in size and here are some of the benefits of this revolutionary cooking appliance:

1. Slow cooker allows cooking delicious and Nutritious meals

Slow cookers can be used to cook fresh ingredients at a low temperature for a long period of time that can reach 8 to 10 hours. This, all the juices and nutritious ingredients of meats will be retained if you use a slow cooker.

2. A time-saver

A slow cooker can save you from slaving over your stove for long hours. All that you need to do to use your slow cooker is to initially prepare your ingredients; toss it together in your slow cooker; then set the timer and do whatever chores you have. When you come back home, you will find your meal ready to serve and enjoy warm.

3. Useful every day in the whole year

Slow cookers are usually associated with wintertime because of its hot dishes and warmth. But, slow cookers can also be used every day of the year anytime you need it. The main perk of using slow cookers during the summer is that it helps you stay away from the stove and oven, two cooking appliances that can make your kitchen really hot and uncomfortable.

4. Slow cookers are energy-saving

Slow-cookers are known for consuming less energy than any conventional cooking appliance like electric oven.

5. A slow cooker is easy- to clean up

Except for a few utensils, a cutting board, a pan for browning the meat, a spoon and a fork; slow cookers are very easy-to clean.

6. Slow cookers are transportable

Slow cookers are characterized by being transportable; it is an appliance that you can pack in your luggage and take it with you wherever you go even in summer holidays.

> **Note**

When shopping for a new slow cooker; you should pay attention to how many people you will be cooking for. You can find small, medium and large-sized slow cookers. Some brands of slow cookers have an inner ceramic interior and some other brands are equipped with an inner cast iron pot that allows you to brown the meat before cooking your meal.

Slow Cooker Times and temperatures

Determining the slow cooker times

Slow cooker recipes need an average cooking time that varies from 6 to 10 hours. So if you want to cook a wide range of your favourite recipes and dishes using a slow cooker, here are some guidelines you can follow:

Slow Cooking Times

To cook a traditional Recipe in a slow cooker; here are the settings you can use:

Traditional Slow cooker Recipe	High setting, Slow Cooker	Low setting, Slow Cooker
45 to 50 minutes	3 to 4 hours	6 to 10 hours
50 to 60 minutes	4 to 5 hours	8 to 10 hours

Slow cooking main temperatures

Make sure to choose a thermometer so that it helps you determine if your dish is perfectly cooked and to help you learn how to adjust the temperature of your slow cooker, here is a simple guide:

Food types	Cooking Temperatures in Degrees F
Egg dishes	160 to 165

Eggs	Cook the eggs until the yolk is firm
Chicken and Turkey	165 to 170
Beef, Veal, pork and lamb	160 to 165
Beef meat	
Medium rare beef meat	140 to 145
Medium cooked beef	160 to 165
Well done meat	170 to 175
Medium rare Lamb	145
Medium cooked lamb	160
Well done lamb	170
Pork	155
Medium cooked pork	160
Well done pork	170
Poultry	
Whole Chicken	180
Whole Turkey	180
Roasted Poultry breasts	170
Wings and Poultry thighs	180
Fresh Ham	160
Precooked Ham	140

Slow cooker tips

If you have recently purchased a slow cooker and you don't know to use it, don't panic, slow cookers are easy-to use, all you have to do is to follow the tips below:

1. Before using your slow cooker for the first time, make sure to remove the lid and the crock insert; then wash it with warm water; then rinse and dry it very well.
2. Always make sure to place the slow cooker over a flat surface or counter.
3. Each recipe has recommended temperature that you can set; some recipes are cooked on Low while others are cooked rather on High. The temperature setting high allows the cooking time to be halved.
4. When you want to cook a certain recipe with vegetables; place it in the crock insert; then place the meat right on top.
5. Make sure that the liquid you use comes half way of the wall of the slow cooker inner crock insert.
6. When you want to roast whole pieces of beef, chicken or lamb; you don't need to add extra liquid. Portions of meat should be barely covered with the liquid in your slow cooker.
7. When cooking meat for casserole recipes; lightly coat the pieces of meat into flour and brown it before adding it to your slow cooker. This process can help retain the flavours and the meat juices within and makes the meat tender.
8. You can place frozen casseroles in slow cooker and heat it for about 5 to 8 hours; but you should remember not to place frozen ingredients directly in your slow cooker.
9. If you notice that a recipe has too much liquid within it; turn your slow cooker to High; then remove the lid on the slow cooker and make sure that enough liquid has evaporated.

10. Always make sure to keep your slow cooker covered and do not remove the lid during the cooking process.
11. Do not use your slow cooker to reheat food; if you want to reheat a certain meal, you can just use the oven to do so.
12. Do not place the crock insert into cold water while it is still hot.
13. You can use the setting 'Warm' to keep your meals, warm when serving it.

Slow cooker Safeguards

To prevent any type of personal property or injury when using a slow cooker; here are some of the most important safeguards and instructions you can follow:

1. When using a slow cooker, there are some precautions you have to pay attention not to touch any knobs or handles and make sure not to touch any hot pads.
2. Always make sure to unplug the slow cooker from the outlet when you are not using it.
3. Always allow the slow cooker to cool before cleaning it and before taking out its parts for cleaning.
4. Make sure to keep the slow cooker out of children's reach.
5. Do never plug your slow cooker with a damages cord; you can risk damaging your cooking appliance.
6. Do not use your slow cooker outdoors.
7. Do not place a slow cooker near an electric burner or in a hot oven.
8. Do not use your slow cooker appliance for any other than its intended use.

9. To protect yourself against an electric shock, try not to immerse the slow cooker cord in water.
10. If, for any reason, you slow cooker doesn't work • Do not attempt to repair this appliance yourself.
11. Do not use a glass cover if over your slow cooker if it has deep scratches, it will end up shattering.
12. Be extremely careful when you remove the cover of the slow cooker; make sure to lift it slowly so that the steam doesn't harm your face.
13. Don't set the slow cooker directly over a table or a counter.
14. If you want to preheat your slow cooker; make sure to preheat it with the cover on.
15. Do not set the hot cover of your slow cooker over a wet surface and let it cool before doing so or before placing it into water.

> **Note:**

After each slow cooker use; make sure to wipe the exterior part of your slow cooker with a clean damp cloth; then dry it. Do not use any chemicals or scourers to clean your slow cooker because it can lead to a serious damage to the surface.

CHAPTER 2: WHOLE30 SLOW COOKER RECIPES

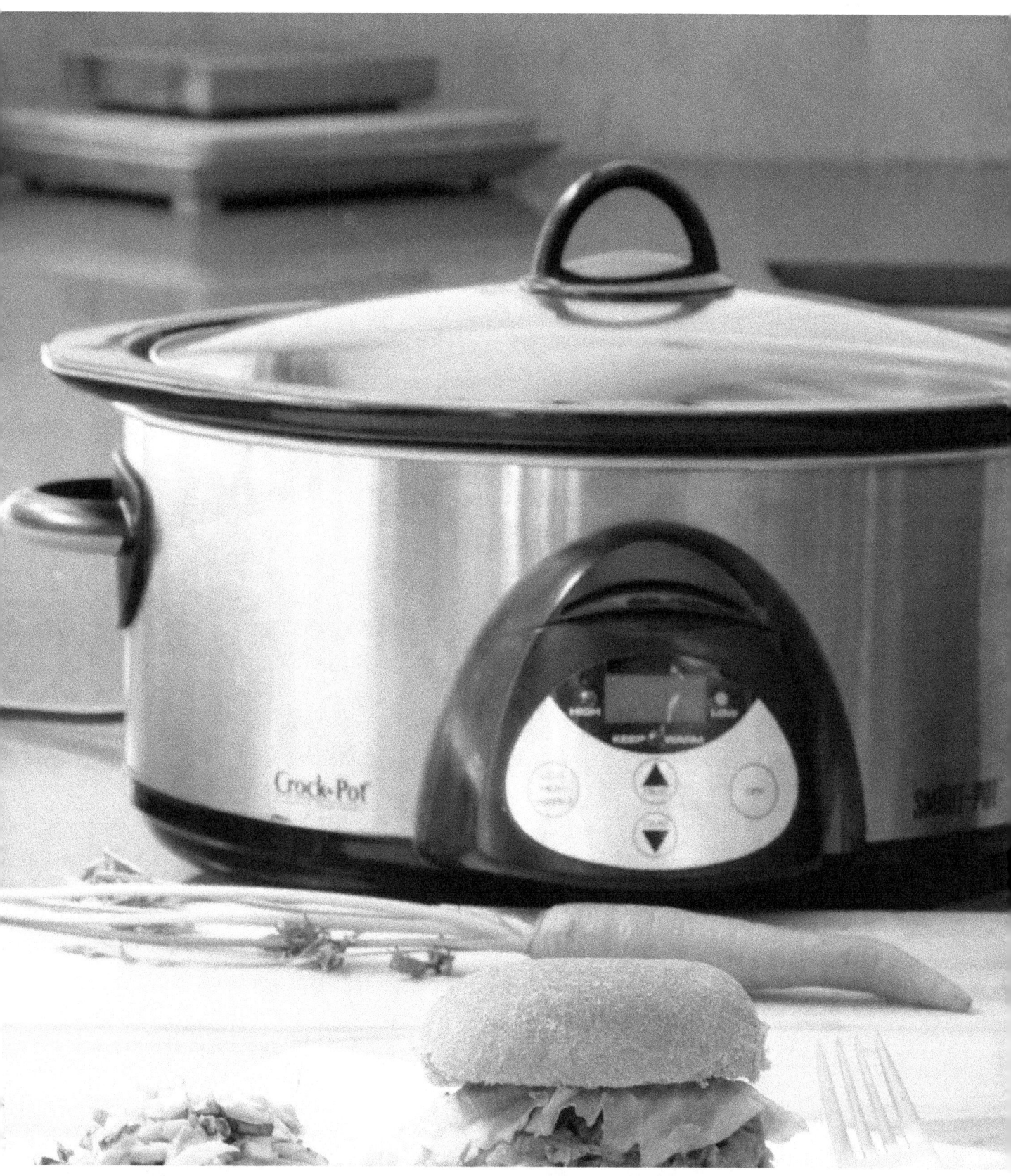

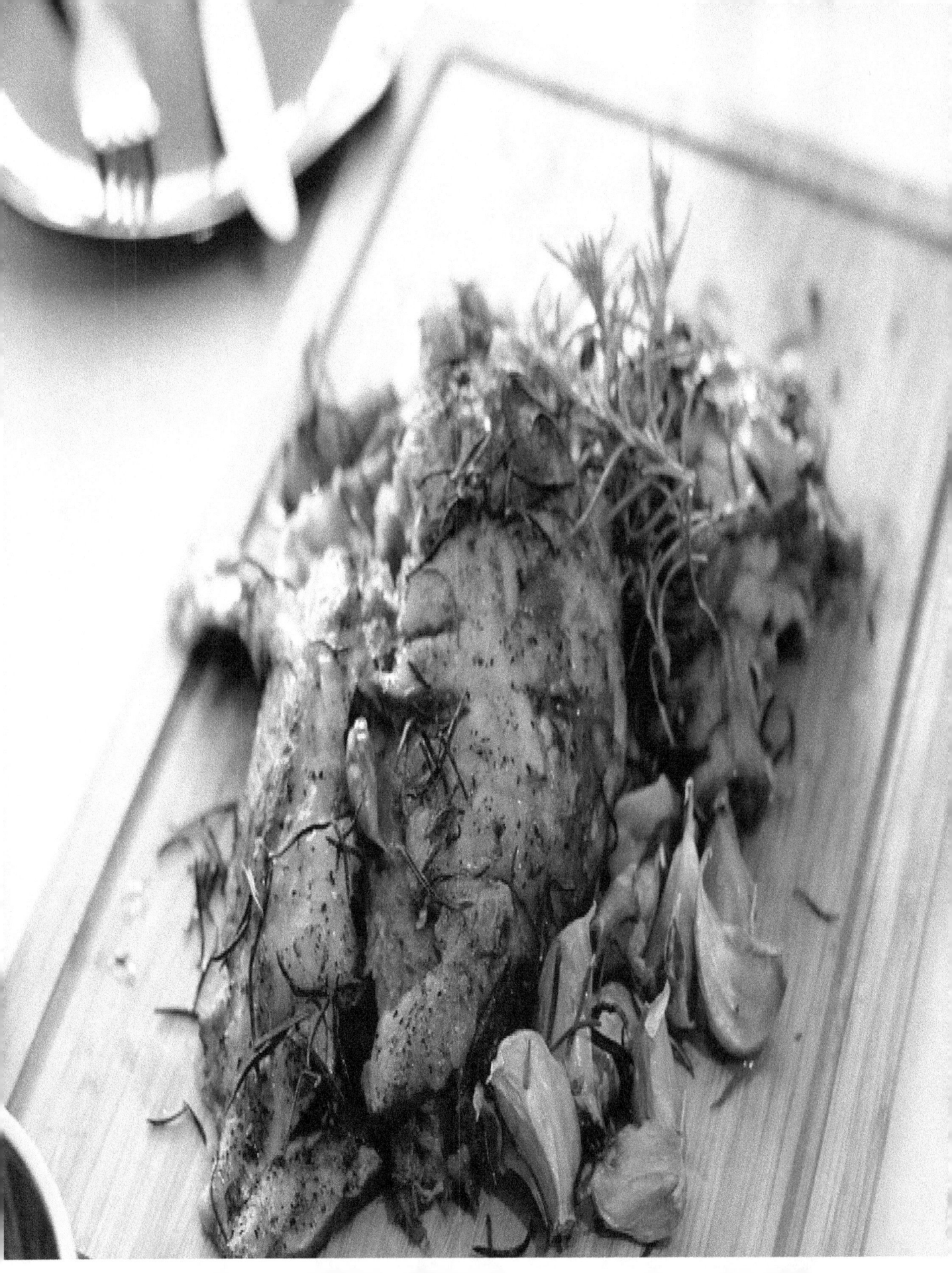

Whole30 Slow Cooker Lamb Recipes

Recipe 1: Rack of lamb with thyme and rosemary

(Prep time: 8 Mins|Cook Time: 8 Hours| Servings: 4)

Ingredients

- 1 and ½ pounds of racks of lamb
- 3 Tablespoons of olive oil
- 2 Tablespoons of chopped fresh rosemary
- 1 Tablespoon of chopped fresh thyme
- ½ Cup of water
- 1 Cup of water
- 1 teaspoon of lemon zest
- 3 Roughly chopped garlic cloves
- 1 Teaspoon of minced root ginger

Instructions

1. Preheat your slow cooker to Low
2. In a large frying pan and over a medium high heat, warm about 1 tablespoon of olive oil in a large skillet and brown it on all sides for about 2 minutes
3. Set the browned meat aside; then combine the remaining ingredients in a large bowl and toss very well
4. Put the lamb in the bottom of your slow cooker; then pour the mixture you have prepared over the lamb and cover the slow cooker with the lid
5. Cook your lamb on Low for about 6 to 8 hours
6. Remove the lid of your slow cooker when the time is up
7. Serve and enjoy your lamb with the juices in the bottom of your slow cooker

8. Serve and enjoy your dish!

Nutrition Information

Calories: 325, Fat: 18g, Carbohydrates: 11.5g, Protein: 35g, Dietary Fiber 3g

Recipe 2: Slow cooked Rolled lamb

(Prep time: 5 Mins|Cook Time: 8 Hours| Servings: 5)

Ingredients

- 5 Crushed garlic cloves
- 2 Tablespoons of freshly squeezed lemon juice
- 3 Tablespoons of chopped, fresh rosemary
- 1 Tablespoon of Dijon mustard
- 2 Teaspoons of olive oil
- 1 and 1/4 teaspoons of kosher salt
- 1 Pinch of fresh ground black pepper
- 3 an ½ pounds of uncooked trimmed boneless, tied and rolled lamb leg.

Instructions

1. Preheat your slow cooker to a low heat; then line it with an aluminium foil
2. Combine the crushed garlic, the rosemary, the lemon juice, the mustard, the olive oil, the salt and the pepper; mix your ingredients very well; then rub the mixture over the lamb
3. With a butcher's twine, roll the lamb and brown it in a large pan and over a medium high heat for about 5 minutes
4. Place the rolled lamb into your slow cooker over the aluminium foil
5. Cover the slow cooker with the lid and cook on Low for about 7 to 8 hours or on High for about 4 hours

6. When the time is up; turn off your slow cooker and remove the lamb; then set it aside to cool for about 15 minutes
7. Slice the lamb into slices of ¼ inch of thickness each
8. Serve and enjoy your dish!

Nutrition Information

Calories: 213, Fat: 9g, Carbohydrates: 1.5g, Protein: 29g, Dietary Fiber 2.3g

Recipe 3: Moroccan style lamb stew

(Prep time: 10 Mins|Cook Time: 8 Hours| Servings: 4)

Ingredients

- 2 Pounds of lamb stew meat, each cut into pieces of 1 inch each
- 1 Chopped onion
- 2 Diced tomatoes
- 2 Peeled and sliced carrots
- 2 Peeled and sliced parsnips
- 9 to 10 dried apricots
- 2 Cups of lamb stock
- 1 tbsp of minced ginger
- 2 Minced garlic cloves
- 1 Tablespoon of ground cumin
- 1 Teaspoon of fennel seeds
- 1 Teaspoon of ground coriander
- ¼ Teaspoon of ground cinnamon
- ¼ tsp of ground allspice
- 1 Cinnamon stick
- ½ Cup of coconut milk
- Chopped fresh cilantro
- 2 Tablespoons of coconut oil
- 1 Pinch of sea salt
- 1 Pinch of freshly ground black pepper

Instructions

1. Preheat your slow cooker to Low
2. In a large pan and over a medium heat, melt the coconut oil in a large skillet; then brown the meat on all its sides for about 1 minute per side
3. Add all the spices, the fennel, the cumin, the coriander, the ground cinnamon and the ground allspice to the lamb and stir very well
4. Place the meat in the bottom of your slow cooker and add in the garlic, the ginger and the chopped onion
5. Add in the carrots, the tomatoes, the parsnips, and the dried apricots to your slow cooker with the coconut milk
6. Pour the lamb stock over your ingredients and top it with the cinnamon stick
7. Cover the slow cooker with a lid and cook on Low for about 6 to 8 hours or on High for about 4 hours
8. When the time is up, turn off your slow cooker
9. Serve and enjoy your dish with chopped fresh cilantro

Nutrition Information

Calories: 264, Fat: 13g, Carbohydrates: 8g, Protein: 14g, Dietary Fiber 1.8g

Recipe 4: Slow cooked Rolled lamb

(Prep time: 10 Mins|Cook Time: 8 Hours| Servings: 4)

Ingredients

- 8 Trimmed, bone in lamb chops
- 3 Crushed garlic cloves
- 1 Teaspoon of extra-virgin olive oil
- ½ Fresh lemons
- 1 and ¼ teaspoon of kosher salt
- 1 Tablespoon of Za'atar
- 1 Pinch of fresh ground pepper

Instructions

1. Preheat your slow cooker on a low heat and spray it with cooking spray
2. Rub the lamb chops with garlic and oil.
3. Squeeze a little bit of lemon juice on both sides of the meat; then season it with 1 pinch of salt and 1 pinch of ground black pepper
4. Brown the lamb in a large skillet over a medium high heat for about 3 minutes per side
5. Transfer the browned meat to the bottom of your slow cooker and cook on Low for about 7 hours or on High for about 3 and ½ hours
6. Serve and enjoy your dish!

Nutrition Information

Calories: 206, Fat: 8g, Carbohydrates: 2g, Protein: 27g, Dietary Fiber 1.2g

Recipe 5: Lamb casserole with spinach and kale

(Prep time: 12 Mins|Cook Time: 5 Hours| Servings: 3-4)

Ingredients

- 2 Cups of lamb stock
- 1 and ½ pounds of diced lamb shoulder
- 1 Bunch of 1 pound of spinach
- 1 Big bunch of 1 pounds of kale with the stems removed
- 2 Tablespoons of coconut oil
- 1 to 2 finely chopped onions
- 1 Inch of grated or minced piece of ginger
- 3 Minced garlic cloves
- 1 long, finely diced green chili
- 1 and ½ teaspoons of sea salt
- 1 and ½ teaspoons of ground coriander

- 1 and ½ teaspoons of ground cumin
- 1 Teaspoon of Garam Masala
- ½ tsp of ground turmeric
- ¼ Teaspoon of cayenne pepper
- ½ tsp of black pepper

Instructions

1. Heat the coconut oil in a pan over a medium high heat; then add in the diced onion and the garlic and cook for about 5 minutes
2. Add the ginger, the peppers and the spices for about 1 minute
3. Pour the stock in a pan over a high heat and cook for about 1 minute
4. Put the lamb in your slow cooker and cook on high for about 4 hours or on Low for 8 hours
5. Bring a large pan of water to boil; then add the spinach and the kale and boil for about 5 minutes
6. Drain the kale and spinach and pulse it together until it becomes smooth; then pour the mixture in your slow cooker and stir
7. Cover your slow cooker with a lid and cook on Low for about 30 minutes
8. Serve and enjoy your dish!

Nutrition Information

Calories: 283, Fat: 12.1g, Carbohydrates: 6g, Protein: 17g, Dietary Fiber 2.5g

Recipe 6: Slow cooked Lamb meatballs

(Prep time: 5 Mins|Cook Time: 6 Hours| Servings: 10)

Ingredients

To make the meatballs

- 2 Pounds of ground lamb
- ¼ Cup of chopped fresh parsley
- 1 Minced garlic clove
- 1 and ½ tbsp of Za'atar seasoning
- 1 Teaspoon of kosher salt
- 3 Tablespoons of water
- 2 Tablespoons of olive oil

To make the gremolata:
- 2 Tbsp of chopped fresh parsley
- 2 Tbsp of chopped fresh mint
- 1 Tbsp of lime zest
- 2 Minced garlic cloves

Instructions

1. To prepare the meatballs, combine all the ingredients except for the oil in a bowl and mix very well
2. Form 24 meatballs from the mixture of the meat
3. Preheat your slow cooker to Low; then spray it with cooking spray
4. Arrange the meatballs in the bottom of your slow cooker and cover the slow cooker with the lid
5. Cook your meatballs for about 3 hours on High or on Low for about 6 hours
6. When the time is up; turn off your slow cooker; then remove the meatballs and place it on paper towels to cool
7. Prepare the gremolata by combining its ingredients very well
8. Serve and enjoy your lamb meatballs with the gremolata!

Nutrition Information

Calories: 305, Fat: 11g, Carbohydrates: 4g, Protein: 34g, Dietary Fiber 2g

Recipe 7: Lamb Curry

(Prep time: 10 Mins|Cook Time: 7 Hours and 30 minutes| Servings: 5)

Ingredients

- 1 Tablespoon of coconut oil
- 1 and ½ pounds of diced lamb
- 1 Large, diced red onion
- ½ long, finely diced red chilli
- 2 Medium, diced celery sticks
- 3 Diced garlic cloves
- 2 and ½ teaspoons of Garam Masala powder
- 1 and ¼ teaspoons of turmeric powder
- 1 teaspoon of fennel seeds
- 1 and ½ teaspoons of coconut oil
- 1 and ½ cups of coconut milk
- 1 and ½ tablespoons of tomato paste
- 1 Cup of water
- 1 and ⅓ teaspoons of sea salt
- 2 Medium, diced carrots
- 1 Squeeze of lemon juice or of lime
- 1 Dash or chopped parsley
- Chopped coriander for garnishing

Instructions

1. Preheat your slow cooker to Low and spray it with cooking spray
2. Heat 1 tablespoon of coconut oil in a large pan over a medium high heat, then add in the lamb and brown it for about 4 minutes
3. Add the chilli, the onion and the celery to your slow cooker; then add the garlic, the Garam Masala, the turmeric, the fennel seeds and the coconut oil
4. Stir your ingredients very well together: then add in the coconut milk, the tomato paste, the water and the sea salt. Stir your ingredients and cover the slow cooker with a lid and cook for ½ hour on Low
5. Add the carrots and cook on Low for about 7 hours or on High for about 3 and ½ hours

6. When the time is up, turn off your slow cooker; then sprinkle some fresh parsley or coriander and drizzle with lime juice or lemon
7. Serve and enjoy your dish!

Nutrition Information

Calories: 273, Fat: 12g, Carbohydrates: 9g, Protein: 31g, Dietary Fiber 2.2g

Recipe 8: Spicy Lamb kheema with peas

(Prep time: 5 Mins|Cook Time: 6 Hours| Servings: 3)

Ingredients
- 1 Minced large onion
- 3 Minced garlic cloves garlic
- 1 Teaspoon of chopped ginger
- 2 Teaspoon of ghee
- 1 Pound of lean ground lamb
- 1 Teaspoon of coriander
- 1 Teaspoon of cumin
- 1 Teaspoon of chili powder
- 1 Teaspoon of turmeric
- 1 Teaspoon of Garam Masala
- 1 Teaspoon of cinnamon
- 1 Cup of frozen peas
- 1 Minced chili pepper
- 2 Tablespoons of chopped fresh cilantro
- ½ Teaspoon of cayenne pepper
- ¼ Cup of tomato sauce
- 1 to 2 bay leaves
- 1 Pinch of salt
- 1 Pinch of fresh ground black pepper

Instructions
1. Preheat your slow cooker to Low

2. Heat the ghee in a large pan over a medium high heat; then add the onions and cook for 5 minutes
3. Add the garlic and the ginger and cook for about 2 minutes
4. Add the ground meat and cook for about 2 minutes
5. Transfer the mixture to the bottom of your slow cooker and season with 1 pinch of salt, 1 pinch of pepper
6. Add the cumin, the coriander, the cayenne, the chili powder, the Tumeric, the Garam Masala and the cinnamon and stir very well
7. Add in the chopped chili pepper, the cilantro, the bay leaf, the tomato sauce and about ½ cup of water
8. Stir very well; then add the peas and cover your slow cooker with the lid; then cook for about 6 hours on Low or for about 3 hours on High
9. When the time is up; turn off your slow cooker
10. Serve and enjoy your dish!

Nutrition Information

Calories: 239.5, Fat: 14g, Carbohydrates: 10g, Protein: 15.8g, Dietary Fiber 2.1g

Recipe 9: Slow cooked lamb with sweet potatoes

(Prep time: 5 Mins|Cook Time: 7 Hours| Servings: 4)

Ingredients

- 2 Tablespoons of olive oil
- 3 to 4 large lean lamb leg chops, about 1 and ¼ pounds
- 2 Chopped, medium onion
- 2 Crushed garlic cloves garlic
- 1 Teaspoon of ground coriander seeds
- 7 Whole, split, cardamom pods
- 1 Small or medium chopped into chunks, sweet potato
- 2 Stock cubes dissolved in about 2 cups of hot water

Instructions

1. Place the lamb, the onions, the garlic, the coriander, the cardamom, the sweet potato and the stock in a 5-Qt slow cooker
2. Season your ingredients with 1 pinch of salt and 1 pinch of ground black pepper
3. Cover your slow cooker with a lid and cook on Low for about 7 Hours or on High for about 3 and ½ hours
4. Serve and enjoy your dish with steamed broccoli!

Nutrition Information
Calories: 348, Fat: 15g, Carbohydrates: 8g, Protein: 25.2g, Dietary Fiber 2.6g

Recipe 10: Lamb Tagine with olives

(Prep time: 7 Mins|Cook Time: 4 Hours| Servings: 5)

Ingredients

- 2 Pounds of cubes lamb shoulder, cut into small cubes
- 1 Dash of saffron
- ¼ teaspoon of ground turmeric
- 1 teaspoon of ground ginger
- ¼ teaspoon of ground cayenne
- ½ Teaspoon of freshly grated black pepper
- ¼ teaspoon of ground cumin
- 1 Pinch of Celtic sea salt
- ¼ Cup of coconut oil
- 1 Diced, large yellow onion
- 1 Bunch of fresh parsley
- 1 Bunch of fresh cilantro
- 1 Cup of drained and pitted green olives

- 1 to 2 Organic fresh lemons
- The juice of 1 lemon

Instructions

1. Mix the dry spices with 1 pinch of salt and add it to your food processor
2. Add in the onion, the parsley and the cilantro and the ground lamb and pulse into small chunks
3. Put the coconut oil, the pulsed mixture of the onion and the spices; then add the ground lamb and the spices in a slow cooker
4. Mix your ingredients with a spoon until the meat is very well combined
5. Cover your slow cooker with its lid and cook your ingredients on low for about 4 hours.
6. Add the pitted olives in the last half hour; then add the lemon juice and season with 1 pinch of salt
7. Serve and enjoy your dish with cauliflower rice!

Nutrition Information

Calories: 214.7, Fat: 11.5g, Carbohydrates: 10g, Protein: 17.8g, Dietary Fiber 2.3g

Whole30 Slow Cooker Pork Recipes

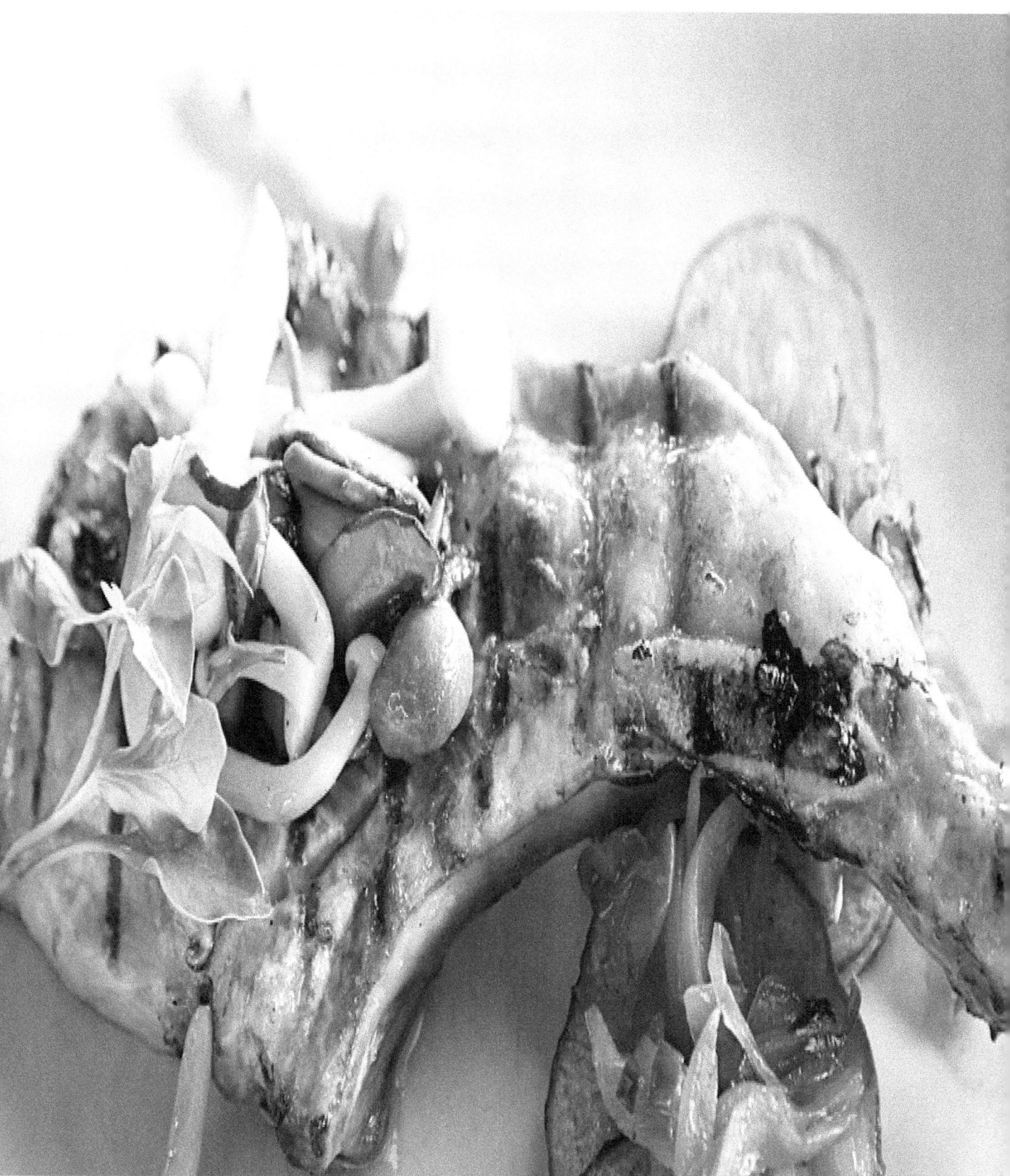

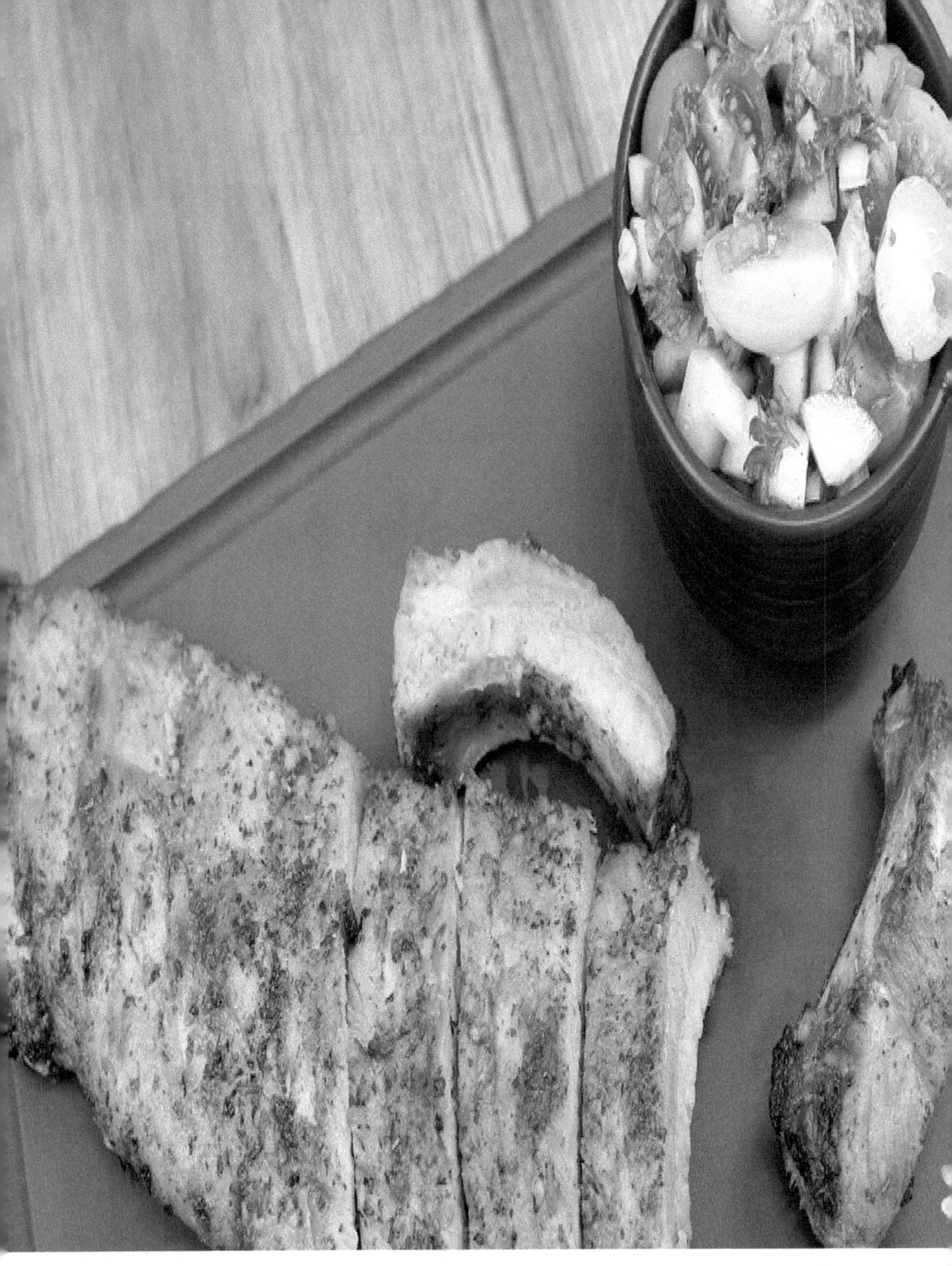

Recipe 11: Spicy pulled pork

(Prep time: 7 Mins|Cook Time: 8 Hours| Servings: 3)

Ingredients

- 3 Pounds of lean pork tenderloin
- 1 Quartered onion
- 4 Sliced garlic cloves
- 4 Whole jalapenos
- 1 Tablespoon of paprika
- 1 Tablespoon of garlic powder
- 1 Tablespoon of chilli powder
- 2 Teaspoon of salt
- 2 Teaspoons of cumin
- 1 Teaspoon of pepper
- 1 Cup of sugar free barbecue sauce
- ½ Cup of low sodium chicken broth

Instructions

1. Mix the spices all together; then rub it over the pork
2. Add the onions, the garlic, and the whole jalapenos to your slow cooker.
3. Put the pork on the top of your veggies in your slow cooker
4. Mix the barbecue sauce with the chicken broth and pour it over the pork
5. Cover your slow cooker with the lid and cook on Low for about 8 hours
6. When the time is up; turn off your slow cooker and shred the meat with two forks; then let the pork rest into the sauce for about 30 minutes
7. Serve and enjoy your spicy pork dish!

Nutrition Information

Calories: 240, Fat: 4g, Carbohydrates: 9g, Protein: 32g, Dietary Fiber 2g

Recipe 12: Pork with orange juice

(Prep time: 5 Mins|Cook Time: 2 Hours| Servings: 4)

Ingredients

- 2 Large apples
- 1 Medium chopped onion
- 4 large, thick diced pork chops
- ½ Cup of sugar-free barbecue sauce
- ¼ Cup of water

Instructions

1. Start by thinly slice the apples and the onions and transfer it to a large bowl of a 4 Qt- slow cooker
2. Toss your ingredients very well and spread it into the bottom of your slow cooker
3. Put the pork chops over the onion and apple mixture and evenly space it apart from each other
4. Whisk the barbecue sauce with water in a bowl; then pour the sauce over the pork chops
5. Cover your slow cooker and cook on High for about 2 hours
6. When the time is up; turn off your slow cooker; then serve and enjoy your dish!

Nutrition Information

Calories: 326, Fat: 9g, Carbohydrates: 11g, Protein: 28.9g, Dietary Fiber 2g

Recipe 13: Ham Chowder

(Prep time: 10 Mins|Cook Time: 4 Hours| Servings: 10)

Ingredients
- 4 Sliced parsnips with the tops cut off
- 1 large peeled and sliced sweet potato
- 1 Cup of chopped onion
- 1 Tablespoon of olive oil
- 4 Minced garlic cloves
- 3 to 4 basil leaves with the stems removed
- 1 Teaspoon of sea salt
- ½ Teaspoon of black pepper
- 1 and ½ cups of chicken broth
- 8 Ounces of diced smoked or ham
- 10 Ounces of almond milk
- 2 Tablespoons of tapioca starch
- 2 Tablespoons of coconut aminos
- 1 Pinch of salt
- Olive oil and herbs for the toppings

Instructions
1. Peel and slice your veggies and place it in your slow cooker
2. Pour the broth in your slow cooker with the basil, the garlic; the olive oil, 1 teaspoon of salt and about ½ teaspoon of pepper
3. Cover your slow cooker with the lid and cook on High for about 2 hours
4. Add the almond milk and stir; then blend the cooked mixture until the mixture becomes creamy
5. Return the remaining ingredients with the chopped ham, the starch and season with salt to your slow cooker and cook on Low for about 1 hour
6. When the time is up; turn off your slow cooker; then ladle the soup into serving bowls and drizzle with oil and herbs
7. Serve and enjoy your chowder!

Nutrition Information
Calories: 254, Fat: 20g, Carbohydrates: 6.4g, Protein: 21g, Dietary Fiber 2.3g

Recipe 14: Cajun pork

(Prep time: 5 Mins|Cook Time: 5 Hours| Servings: 4)

Ingredients
- 4 to 5 pork chops
- 1 Small, diced yellow onion
- 1 Cup of sliced mushrooms
- 2 Minced garlic cloves
- 1 and ½ cups of chicken stock
- 1 Cup of coconut milk
- 1 Tablespoon of Cajun seasoning
- 1 Teaspoon of smoked paprika
- 1 Tablespoon of coconut oil
- 1Pinch of sea salt
- 1 Pinch of freshly ground black pepper

Instructions
1. Preheat your slow cooker to Low; then season the pork chops with 1 pinch of salt and 1 pinch of freshly ground black pepper.
2. Melt the coconut oil in a large skillet over a medium high heat and brown the pork chops for about 2 to 3 minutes per side
3. Add the garlic and the onion to the skillet and cook the mixture for about 2 minutes
4. Transfer the mixture to your slow cooker and add in the mushrooms; then pour in the chicken stock
5. Sprinkle in the Cajun seasoning to your slow cooker and season with 1 pinch of salt and the smoked paprika
6. Add the pork chops to your slow cooker
7. Cover the slow cooker with the lid and cook on High for about 2 and ½ hours or for about 5 hours on Low
8. When the time is up; turn off your slow cooker and pour in the coconut milk; give a good stir
9. Serve and enjoy your dish warm!

Nutrition Information
Calories: 234.9, Fat: 8.6g, Carbohydrates: 3g, Protein: 35g, Dietary Fiber 1.4g

Recipe 15: Pork Chili

(Prep time: 10 Mins|Cook Time: 7 Hours| Servings: 4)

Ingredients

- 4 and ¼ pounds of boneless pork shoulder with the fat removed
- 2 Finely sliced onions
- 2 Seeded and finely diced red chillies
- 2 Sliced bell peppers
- 4 Minced garlic cloves
- 1 Can of 28 Oz of diced tomatoes
- ¼ cup of chilli powder;
- 2 tbsp of smoked paprika;
- 1 tbsp of ground cumin;
- ¼ tsp of ground cayenne pepper
- 1 Bunch of minced fresh oregano leaves
- 3 Tablespoons of red vinegar;
- ¼ Cup of extra-virgin olive oil
- 1 Pinch of sea salt
- 1 Pinch of freshly ground black pepper to taste

Instructions

1. Preheat your slow cooker to Low
2. Warm the oil in a large pan over a medium high heat; then add in the garlic, the onions and the red chillies
3. Cook for about 4 minutes; then reduce the heat and add in the diced tomatoes, the bell peppers, the chilli powder, the smoked paprika, the cumin, the cayenne pepper, the oregano leaves, the salt and the pepper and mix very well
4. Add the pork shoulder and stir; then transfer all the mixture of the ingredients to your slow cooker
5. Pour in the red vinegar and add enough water to cover the pork chops
6. Cover the slow cooker with a lid and cook for about 3 and ½ hours on High or 7 hours on Low

7. When the time is up; turn off your slow cooker
8. Serve and enjoy your dish!

Nutrition Information

Calories: 180, Fat: 6.1g, Carbohydrates: 12g, Protein: 13.2g, Dietary Fiber 3.5g

Recipe 16: Slow cooked pork chops with chipotle

(Prep time: 8 Mins|Cook Time: 6 Hours| Servings: 5)

Ingredients

- 4 to 5 Boneless Pork Chops inches of about 1 inch of thickness each
- 2 Tablespoons of olive oil
- To prepare the rub:
- 1 Tablespoon of chili powder
- 1 Teaspoon of paprika
- ½ Teaspoon of cumin
- ½ Teaspoon of chipotle chili pepper spice
- ½ Teaspoon of coarse sea salt
- 1 Minced garlic clove

To prepare the sauce:
- 1 Cup of canned coconut milk
- ½ teaspoon of chipotle chili pepper spice
- 1 Teaspoon of liquid smoke
- ¼ Cup of chopped fresh cilantro
- To make the garnish:
- The juice of 1 lime
- 2Tablespoons of Chopped fresh cilantro

Instructions

1. Preheat your slow cooker to Low; then prepare the pork by mixing the ingredients of the marinade
2. Rub the pork chops with the marinade, the spices and the olive oil

3. Heat a little bit of olive oil in a large skillet and brown the pork in the skillet for about 3 minutes
4. Spray your slow cooker with cooking spray; then transfer the pork meat to your slow cooker
5. Cover your slow cooker with the lid and cook on High for about 3 hours or on Low for about 6 hours
6. While the pork is cooking, mix all together the coconut milk, the chipotle pepper, the cilantro, and the liquid smoke in a food processor and process the mixture until it becomes smooth.
7. Once the time is up; turn off your slow cooker; then pour the sauce over the pork and stir
8. Garnish your dish with the juice of 1 lime and with chopped cilantro
9. Serve and enjoy your dish!

Nutrition Information

Calories: 152.5, Fat: 7.2g, Carbohydrates: 2g, Protein: 21g, Dietary Fiber 1g

Recipe 17: Pork Carnitas

(Prep time: 10 Mins|Cook Time: 8 Hours| Servings: 3)

Ingredients

- 1 Tablespoon of dried oregano
- 2 Teaspoons of ground cumin
- 1 Tablespoon of avocado oil
- 2 Pounds of loin or pork tenderloin
- ½ Chopped onions
- 3 Minced garlic cloves
- 1 Chopped jalapeño
- 2 Teaspoons of salt
- The juice of 1 lime
- The juice of one navel orange
- 1 Tablespoon of avocado oil

Instructions

1. Pat the pork tenderloin dry with clean paper towels; then combine the rub ingredients and rub the tenderloin with it
2. Place the meat in a slow cooker; then top it with the remaining ingredients and cover your slow cooker with a lid
3. Cook your food on high for about 4 to 6 hours on High or for about 6 to 8 hours on Low.
4. When the time is up; turn off your slow cooker and shred the pork with two forks
5. Heat a little bit of olive oil in a large skillet over a medium high heat; then add enough quantity of carnitas and cook for about 5 minutes
6. Cook for about 3 minutes
7. Serve and enjoy your dish!

Nutrition Information

Calories: 221, Fat: 9.1g, Carbohydrates: 3.4g, Protein: 31g, Dietary Fiber 0.3g

Recipe 18: Cuban-style pulled pork

(Prep time: 6 Mins|Cook Time: 8 Hours| Servings: 3)

Ingredients

- 3 Pounds of boneless lean pork shoulder roast, with the fat removed
- 6 Garlic cloves
- 2/3 Cup of grapefruit juice
- The juice of 1 lime
- ½ Tablespoon of fresh oregano
- 1/2 Tablespoon of cumin

- 1 Tablespoon of kosher salt
- 1 to 2 bay leaves
- 2 to 3 lime wedges
- Chopped fresh cilantro
- 1 Cup of hot sauce

Instructions

1. Chop the pork into about 4 pieces
2. Pulse the garlic, the grapefruit juice, the lime juice, the oregano, the cumin and the very well with a blender
3. Pour the prepared marinade over the pork pieces and set it aside for about 1 hour
4. Transfer the marinated pork to your slow cooker; then add the bay leaf and cover your slow cooker with a lid
5. Cook on Low for about 8 hours; then remove the pork and shred it with two forks
6. Remove the liquid from your slow cooker; the return it to your slow cooker
7. Add in about 1 cup of the liquid you have removed back to your slow cooker and season with 1 pinch of salt
8. Cook on Low for about ½ hours
9. Serve and enjoy your dish!

Nutrition Information

Calories: 213, Fat: 10.5g, Carbohydrates: 2.7g, Protein: 26g, Dietary Fiber 0.52g

Recipe 19: Pork with orange juice

(Prep time: 10 Mins|Cook Time: 4 Hours| Servings: 3)

Ingredients

- 1 Tablespoon of coconut oil
- 2 Coarsely chopped garlic cloves

- 1 and ½ pounds of boneless pork loin
- 1 tablespoon of kosher Salt
- ½ Teaspoon of freshly ground pepper
- ½ Teaspoon of dried Italian seasoning
- 1 to 2 rosemary, chopped sprig leaves
- ¾ Cup of fresh squeezed orange juice
- ¾ Cup of low sodium chicken stock

Instructions

1. Preheat your slow cooker to Low and spray it with cooking spray
2. Sprinkle the salt, the pepper, the chopped rosemary and the Italian seasoning over both sides of the pork
3. Use a butcher twine to tie the pork loin together
4. In a large skillet, heat the oil; then add the pork and brown the meat for about 4 minutes with the fat side down
5. Add in the garlic and cook for about 2 to 3 minutes
6. Pour in the stock and the orange juice and let boil on a low heat for about 7 minutes
7. Transfer your ingredients into your slow cooker
8. Cover your slow cooker with a lid and cook on Low for about 6 hours or on High for about 3 hours
9. When the time is up, transfer the pork to a cutting board to rest; then slice the slow cooked pork and let rest for about 5 minutes
10. Slice the pork meat; then serve and enjoy your pork!

Nutrition Information

Calories: 165, Fat: 7g, Carbohydrates: 3g, Protein: 21g, Dietary Fiber 0.1g

Recipe 20: Pork patties

(Prep time: 5 Mins|Cook Time: 4 Hours| Servings: 10)

Ingredients

- 1 Pound of ground pork
- 1 Crushed garlic clove
- ½ Teaspoon of paprika
- ½ Teaspoon of chilli flakes
- ½ Teaspoon of sage
- 1 Pinch of ground cloves
- ½ Cup of shredded apple
- ¼ Teaspoon of salt
- ¼ Teaspoon of pepper

Instructions

1. Preheat your slow cooker to Low and spray it with cooking spray
2. Combine the ingredients of the pork with your hands and mix everything together very well
3. Make the shape of 10 patties from the mixture
4. Arrange the patties into the bottom of your slow cooker
5. Cover the slow cooker with the lid and cook on Low for about 4 hours or on High for about 2 hours
6. When the time is up; turn off your slow cooker
7. Serve and enjoy your pork patties.

Nutrition Information

Calories: 101, Fat: 8g, Carbohydrates: 3g, Protein: 11.8g, Dietary Fiber 1.5g

Whole30 Slow Cooker Beef Recipes

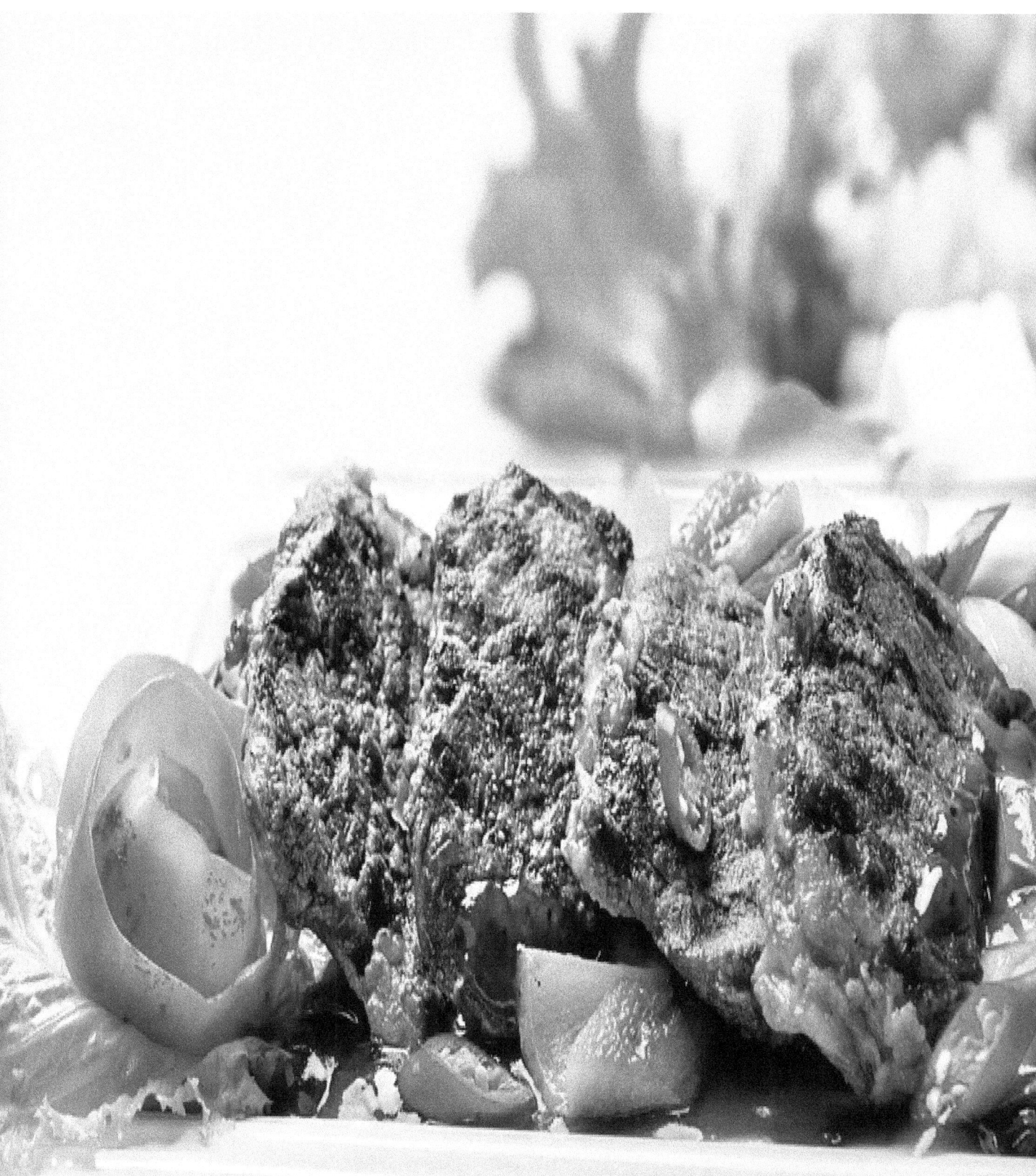

Recipe 21: Beef with broccoli

(Prep time: 7 Mins|Cook Time: 2 Hours| Servings: 4-5)

Ingredients

- 1 Pound of grass-fed sliced steak
- 1 Cup of broth or beef stock
- 4 Minced garlic cloves garlic
- 1/8 Teaspoon of grated ginger
- 1/3 Cup of coconut aminos
- 1 Tablespoon of avocado oil
- ¼ Teaspoon of red pepper flakes
- 12 Ounces of fresh or frozen broccoli
- ½ Teaspoon of xanthan gum

Instructions

1. Preheat your slow cooker to Low and spray it with cooking spray
2. Place the steak in your slow cooker with the beef stock, the garlic, the ginger, the coconut aminos, the oil and the red pepper flakes
3. Cook your meal on Low for about 2 to 3 hours
4. When the time is up; turn off your slow cooker
5. Sprinkle the xanthan gum on top
6. Stir in the broccoli florets and cook on Low for about ½ hour
7. Serve and enjoy your dish!

Nutrition Information

Calories: 323, Fat: 19g, Carbohydrates: 11g, Protein: 26g, Dietary Fiber 2g

Recipe 22: Slow cooked ground beef casserole with cabbage

(Prep time: 5 Mins|Cook Time: 7 Hours| Servings: 5-6)

Ingredients

To make the meatballs:
- 1 and ¾ pounds of 85% lean ground beef
- 1 Pasteurized egg
- ¾ Teaspoon of fine grain sea salt
- 2 Teaspoon of onion powder
- ½ Teaspoon of garlic powder
- 1 Tablespoon of Italian seasoning blend
- 1 Pinch of crushed red pepper
- 1 Tablespoon of chopped fresh parsley
- To make the sauce:
- 1 Can of 28 Oz of crushed tomatoes with basil
- 1 Can of 14 Oz of diced tomatoes with garlic and basil and garlic
- 1 Can of 6 Oz of tomato paste
- ½ medium chopped onions
- 2 Tablespoons of chopped fresh garlic
- 2 tbsp chopped fresh oregano leaves
- 2 bay leaves
- 1 Pinch of sea salt to taste

Instructions

1. Preheat your slow cooker to Low and spray it with cooking spray
2. Start by preparing the meatballs and to do that mix the garlic powder with the salt, the Italian seasoning and the crushed red pepper
3. In a medium bowl, add in the ground beef and sprinkle it with 1 pinch of salt
4. Add in the pasteurized egg and gently combine the mixture with both your hands
5. Add more parsley and mix again
6. Arrange the meatballs in the bottom of your slow cooker
7. Top the beef meatballs with the ingredients of the sauce and stir

8. Cover your slow cooker with the lid and cook on Low for about 4 hours on Low
9. When the time is up; turn off your slow cooker
10. Serve and enjoy your meal!

Nutrition Information

Calories: 186, Fat: 10g, Carbohydrates: 3.2g, Protein: 26g, Dietary Fiber 1.2g

Recipe 23: Slow cooked ground beef casserole with cabbage

(Prep time: 5 Mins|Cook Time: 7 Hours| Servings: 3-4)

Ingredients

- ½ Roughly sliced cabbage
- 1 Diced onion
- 3 Finely chopped garlic cloves
- 1 and ½ pounds of ground beef
- 1 and ½ cups of crushed tomatoes
- 2 Cups of cauliflower rice
- 4 Tablespoons of coconut oil
- 1 Heaping tablespoon of Italian Seasoning
- 1/2 Teaspoon of crushed red pepper
- 1 Pinch of salt
- 1 Pinch of freshly ground pepper
- ½ Cup of finely chopped fresh parsley

Instructions

1. Stir all together your ingredients except for the fresh parsley in a 7- quart slow cooker and stir

2. Cover your slow cooker with a lid and cook on Low for about 7 hours on Low or for about 3 and ½ to 4 hours on High
3. When the time is up; turn off your slow cooker
4. Serve your dish in serving plates and top it with fresh parsley
5. Serve and enjoy your meal!

Nutrition Information

Calories: 302, Fat: 21g, Carbohydrates: 9g, Protein: 18.3g, Dietary Fiber 3g

Recipe 24: Spicy Beef Chilli

(Prep time: 5 Mins|Cook Time: 6 Hours| Servings: 3)

Ingredients

- 2 Pounds of ground beef
- 1 Medium, diced onion
- 3 Minced garlic cloves
- 1 Diced green and red pepper
- 1 Cup of finely diced carrots
- 1 Cup of diced celery
- 1 Minced jalapeno
- 1 Can of 28 ounces of crushed tomatoes
- 1 Can of 14 ounces of diced tomatoes
- 1 Can of 15 ounces of tomato sauce
- 3 Tablespoons of chilli powder
- 1 Tablespoon of oregano
- 1 Tablespoon of basil
- 2 Teaspoon of cumin
- 1 Teaspoon of salt
- 1 Teaspoon of pepper
- 1 Teaspoon of onion powder
- ½ Teaspoon of cayenne

- 2 Medium diced avocados

Instructions

1. Sauté the onions and the garlic together in a large pan over a medium high heat
2. Add in the ground beef and brown the meat for about 3 minutes
3. Drain any excess fat; then transfer the mixture of the onion and beef to a slow cooker
4. Add all the vegetables and season with the spices; then stir and cover your slow cooker with its lid
5. Set your slow cooker to Low and cook for about 6 hours
6. When the time is up; turn off your slow cooker
7. Ladle your meal into serving bowls and garnish it with avocado slices
8. Serve and enjoy your beef chilli!

Nutrition Information

Calories: 173.1, Fat: 6.5g, Carbohydrates: 10.6g, Protein: 12g, Dietary Fiber 1.1g

Recipe 25: Barbecue beef with cabbage Coleslaw

(Prep time: 8 Mins|Cook Time: 10 Hours| Servings: 4)

Ingredients

- 2 and ½ pounds of boneless beef chuck roast
- 1 large, thinly sliced yellow onion
- 3 Small diced tomatoes
- 2 Tbsp of Dijon mustard
- 1 and ½ tablespoons of apple cider vinegar
- ½ Cup of water
- 2 Teaspoons of garlic powder
- 1 and ½ teaspoons of dried oregano
- 2 Teaspoons of chilli powder
- 2 Teaspoons of smoked paprika

- 1 Teaspoon of sea salt
- ½ Teaspoon of black pepper
- The ingredients of the Cole slaw

Simple Cole Slaw
- 1 bag of 9 ounces of shredded carrots, green cabbage and red cabbage
- ⅓ Cup of Whole30-compliant mayonnaise made with pasteurized eggs
- 3 Tablespoons of apple cider vinegar
- ¼ Teaspoon of garlic powder
- 1 Pinch of salt
- 1 Pinch of pepper

Instructions

1. Slice the onions and place it in the bottom of your slow cooker.
2. Cut the beef roast into about 3 chunks of about 1 pound each
3. Sear the portions of beef in a little bit of coconut oil for about 4 minutes per side in a large and heavy frying pan
4. Transfer the browned meat to your slow cooker; then add the onion to it and mix very well
5. Combine the rest of your ingredients and add it to your slow cooker; stir again; then cover your slow cooker with the lid and cook for about 8 to 10 hours on Low
6. Remove the meat from your slow cooker to a baking tray and shred it with 2 forks; then return the meat to your slow cooker and stir into the onion
7. Serve your barbecue beef with coleslaw and enjoy its delicious taste!

Nutrition Information

Calories: 325, Fat: 24g, Carbohydrates: 4.3g, Protein: 34g, Dietary Fiber 2g

Recipe 26: Beef stew

(Prep time: 8 Mins|Cook Time: 4 Hours| Servings: 3)

Ingredients

- 2 and 1/2 pounds of cubed beef for stew
- 3 Tablespoons of olive oil
- 2 Pieces of minced, sugar-free Whole30-approved bacon
- 1 Minced onion
- 3 Finely minced garlic cloves
- ¼ Teaspoon of nutmeg
- ¼ Teaspoon of ginger
- ¼ Teaspoon of clove
- ¼ Cup of pine nuts
- ¼ Cup of dried currants
- 1 Tablespoon of capers
- ½ Cup of chopped spinach
- 3 Tablespoons of minced parsley
- 2 Cups of beef stock
- 1 Tablespoon of red vinegar

Instructions

1. Preheat your slow cooker to Low and spray it with cooking spray
2. Heat a little bit of oil in a large pan and brown the beef for about 5 minutes
3. Add the sugar-free bacon to the pan and cook for about 3 minutes
4. Transfer your browned ingredients to your slow cooker and pour in the stock
5. Cover your slow cooker with a lid and cook on High for about 1 and ½ hours or on Low for about 3 hours
6. After about 1 hour, remove the lid of your slow cooker and add in the spinach and cook on Low for about 30 additional minutes

7. Add in the nuts, the currants, the capers, the parsley and the vinegar; stir your ingredients very well and adjust the seasoning
8. Serve and enjoy your meal!

Nutrition Information

Calories: 230, Fat: 29g, Carbohydrates: 6g, Protein: 16g, Dietary Fiber 3.6g

Recipe 27: Beef with mango

(Prep time: 10 Mins|Cook Time: 5 Hours| Servings: 4)

Ingredients

- 3 Pounds of diced grass-fed stew
- 1 Chopped large onion
- 2 Peeled and chopped large mangoes
- 2 Tablespoons of dried Rosemary
- 1 Tablespoon of dried garlic flakes
- 1 Cup of water
- 1 Teaspoon of pink Himalayan salt
- 1 Tablespoon of balsamic vinegar

Instructions

1. Start by chopping the onion and cut it into half; then thinly slice it
2. Chop the mangoes into small pieces
3. Place the meat, the onion, the mangoes, the rosemary, the garlic and the water in your slow cooker and turn it to Low
4. Cook your meal on Low for about 8 hours or on High for about 4 to 5 hours
5. Mix in about 1 tsp of sea salt and 1 tablespoon of balsamic vinegar

6. Stir your meal very well
7. Serve and enjoy your beef meal!

Nutrition Information

Calories: 173.1, Fat: 6.5g, Carbohydrates: 10.6g, Protein: 12g, Dietary Fiber 1.1g

Recipe 28: Shepherd's Pie

(Prep time: 12 Mins|Cook Time: 5 Hours| Servings: 5)

Ingredients

- 1 Pound of ground beef
- 1 Cup of diced carrots
- 1 Medium diced onion
- 1 Cup of diced celery
- 2 to 3 Minced garlic cloves
- 1 Cup of beef broth
- 1 Can of 6 Oz of tomato paste
- 1 Teaspoon of dried thyme
- 1 Teaspoon of salt
- ½ Teaspoon of black pepper
- 3 Medium sweet potatoes
- 2 Teaspoons of avocado oil

Instructions

1. Start by placing the beef to your slow cooker and turn on the slow cooker to High
2. Chop your vegetables and add it to the slow cooker; then pour in the beef broth
3. Add the tomato paste, the thyme, ½ teaspoon of salt, and about ¼ teaspoon of pepper.

4. Mix your ingredients very well and cover the slow cooker with a lid; then cook for about 3 to 4 hours on Low.
5. Wash the sweet potatoes and pierce it with a fork; then microwave it for about 8 minutes
6. Peel the sweet potatoes when it is cool and place it in a bowl with a little bit of oil
7. Season the potatoes with 1 pinch of salt and 1 pinch of pepper
8. Mash the sweet potatoes with a fork of and spoon the mixture over the beef mixture in your slow cooker
9. Spoon the mixture of the potato into your slow cooker and spread it over the meat; then replace the lid; then let cook for about 1 additional hour
10. Serve and enjoy your meal!

Nutrition Information

Calories: 230, Fat: 13g, Carbohydrates: 7g, Protein: 28g, Dietary Fiber 2.7g

Recipe 29: Beef Picadillo

(Prep time: 7 Mins|Cook Time: 2 Hours| Servings: 4-5)

Ingredients

- 1 and ½ pounds of lean ground beef
- ½ Medium; chopped onion
- 2 Minced garlic cloves
- 1 Chopped tomato
- 1 Teaspoon of kosher salt
- ½ Finely chopped red bell pepper
- 2 Tablespoons of cilantro
- ½ Can of 4 oz of tomato sauce
- 1 Teaspoon of ground cumin
- 1 to 2 bay leaves
- 2 Tablespoons of green olives or capers

Instructions

1. Preheat your slow cooker to Low
2. Season the meat with pepper and salt
3. In a large skillet and over a medium high heat, brown the meat for about 3 minutes
4. Transfer the browned meat to your slow cooker
5. Add the onion, the garlic, the tomato and the salt
6. Add the olives of capers, the cumin and the bay leaf; then add in the tomato sauce and about 3 tablespoons of water
7. Cover your slow cooker with a lid and cook for about 2 hours on High
8. When the time is up; turn off your slow cooker
9. Serve and enjoy your succulent beef dish!

Nutrition Information

Calories: 207.1, Fat: 8.6g, Carbohydrates: 5g, Protein: 23g, Dietary Fiber 1.2g

Recipe 30: Slow cooked short beef ribs

(Prep time: 4 Mins|Cook Time: 8 Hours| Servings: 5-6)

Ingredients

- 5 Pounds of grass-fed beef short ribs
- 5 Medium chopped tomatoes
- 1 Medium chopped white onion
- 2 Tablespoons of 1 chopped fresh peach
- 2 Tablespoons of apple cider vinegar
- 2 Tablespoons of dried rosemary
- 1 Tablespoon of Herbs of Provence Spice

- 1 Teaspoon of sea salt
- ½ Teaspoon of ground black pepper
- 9 to 10 fresh basil leaves

Instructions

1. Put all your ingredients except for the beef ribs in a food processor and process for a few minutes
2. Transfer the processed mixture into your slow cooker
3. Add the beef ribs to your slow cooker
4. Turn your slow cooker to Low and cook for about 8 hours
5. When the time is up turn off your slow cooker
6. Serve and enjoy your beef ribs with a salad and toppings of your choice!

Nutrition Information

Calories: 131, Fat: 11.2g, Carbohydrates: 2.3g, Protein: 10g, Dietary Fiber 0.51g

Whole30 Slow Cooker Seafood Recipes

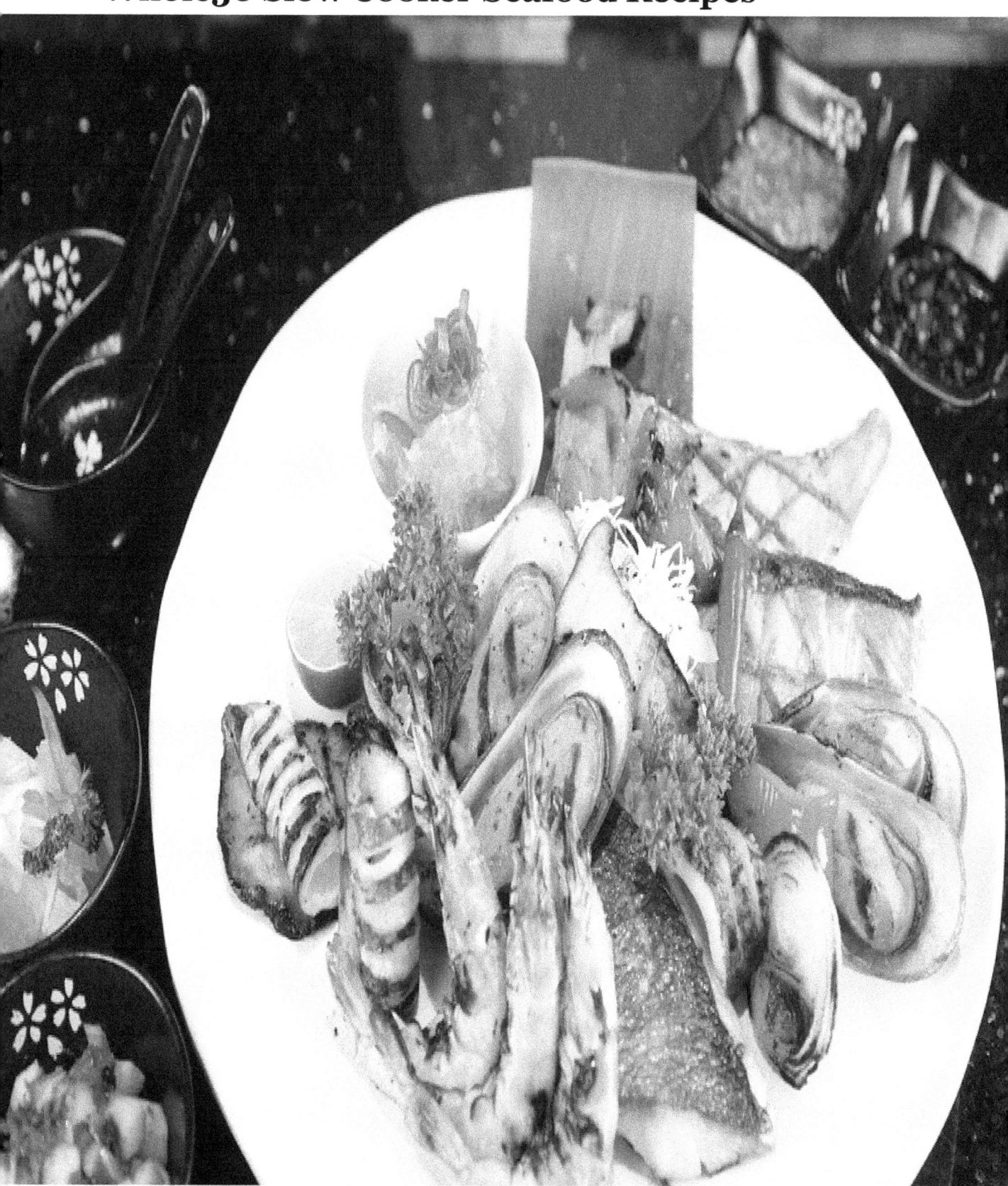

Recipe 31: Fish Curry with coconut milk

(Prep time: 10 Mins|Cook Time: 5 Hours| Servings: 4)

Ingredients

- 1 Pound of Bigeye Jack
- 2 Cups of Coconut Milk
- 2 Diced tomatoes
- 4 Pieces of thinly sliced Jalapeno Peppers
- 1 Piece of thinly sliced Shallot
- 1 Crushed garlic Bulb
- 1 Piece of 2-inch thinly sliced ginger
- 2 Cups of chopped okra
- 1 Piece of chopped carrot
- 1 Teaspoon of Fenugreek Seeds
- 1 Stick of cinnamon
- 1 Teaspoon of Coriander Seeds
- 3 to 4 Pieces of Star Anise
- ½ Teaspoon of Cumin Seeds
- ½ Teaspoon of Mustard Seeds
- 2 Pieces of Bay Leaf
- 3 Tablespoons of Curry Powder

Instructions

1. Gut the fish and scale it; then heat the oil in a wok and toast the cinnamon, the fenugreek, the coriander seeds, the star anise, the cumin seeds and the mustard seeds for about 1 to 2 minutes
2. Add the shallots, the garlic, the ginger, the jalapenos, and the tomatoes and sauté for about 1 minute.
3. Add the curry powder and cook for about 1 additional minute
4. Transfer your mixture to your slow cooker and pour in the coconut milk
5. Cover the slow cooker with its lid and cook on Low for about 4 hours on Low
6. When the time is up; turn off your slow cooker and turn the heat to high

7. Add the fish and cook for about 1 additional hour
8. Season with 1 pinch of salt and pepper
9. Serve and enjoy the fish dish!

Nutrition Information

Calories: 364, Fat: 21.1g, Carbohydrates: 11g, Protein: 22g, Dietary Fiber 3.4g

Recipe 32: Spicy Garlicky Octopus

(Prep time: 5 Mins|Cook Time: 10 Hours| Servings: 3-4)

Ingredients

- 1 Coarsely chopped yellow onion
- 3 Peeled and crushed garlic cloves peeled
- 1 to 2 large bay leaves
- ½ Teaspoons of smoked Spanish paprika
- 1 and ½ teaspoons of kosher salt
- 1 tablespoon of olive oil
- ½ Cup of water
- 1 Pound of Spanish octopus
- 2 Tablespoons of olive oil
- 1/3 Cup of braising liquid
- 1 Tablespoon of fresh lemon juice
- 1 Tablespoon of extra-virgin olive oil
- 1 Pinch of salt
- 1 Pinch of cayenne pepper

Instructions

1. Place the chopped onion, the garlic cloves, the bay leaf, the paprika, the salt, and 1 tablespoon of olive oil into a slow cooker

2. Add the water; then toss in the octopus and cover your slow cooker with a lid
3. Cook for about 8 to 10 hours on Low
4. When the time is up; turn off your slow cooker
5. Stir in the lemon juice, the extra-virgin olive oil, the parsley, the salt, and the cayenne pepper
6. Serve and enjoy your meal!

Nutrition Information

Calories: 299, Fat: 15g, Carbohydrates: 12.1g, Protein: 34g, Dietary Fiber 1.8g

Recipe 33: Spicy Salmon with dill

(Prep time: 6 Mins|Cook Time: 1-2 Hours| Servings: 3)

Ingredients

- 1 to 2 Pounds of salmon
- 2 Minced garlic cloves
- 1 Handful of fresh dill
- 1 Sliced lemon
- 1 Pinch of salt
- 1 Pinch of pepper
- ½ Teaspoon of olive oil

Instructions

1. Line a 4 quart slow cooker with a parchment paper.
2. Season the salmon with 1 pinch of salt, 1 pinch of pepper, the garlic, and the fresh dill.
3. Lay the salmon over the parchment paper
4. Top the salmon with the lemon slices and the oil

5. Cover your slow cooker with a lid and cook on HIGH for about 1 to 2 hours.
6. When the time is up; turn off your slow cooker
7. Serve and enjoy your salmon dish!

Nutrition Information

Calories: 199.1, Fat: 8.2g, Carbohydrates: 2g, Protein: 29.1g, Dietary Fiber 0.2g

Recipe 34: Slow cooked Seafood gumbo

(Prep time: 6 Mins|Cook Time: 5 Hours| Servings: 4)

Ingredients

- 5 Cups of chicken broth
- ¼ Cup of arrowroot flour
- 1 Pound of peeled and deveined raw shrimp with the tails removed
- 2 Pounds of boneless skinless chicken thighs
- 1 Diced onion
- 1 Diced bell pepper
- 3 Diced celery stalks
- 4 Peeled and smashed garlic cloves
- 2 Bay leaves
- 1 Tablespoon of Cajun seasoning mix
- 2 Teaspoons of dried thyme
- 1 Can of diced tomatoes; about 4.5 oz
- ½ Pound of sliced pre-cooked sausages
- 4 Diced green onions

Instructions

1. Mix all together the chicken broth with the arrowroot flour until there are no lumps remaining and set it aside.
2. Chop the onion, the bell pepper, the celery; then peel and smash the garlic.

3. Place the chicken in the bottom of your slow cooker and add in the onion, the bell pepper, the celery, the garlic, and the bay leaves.
4. Sprinkle the Cajun seasoning and the thyme on top.
5. Pour in the chicken broth; the diced tomatoes and the chicken broth; then cook on Low for about 8 hours or on High for about 4 hours.
6. When there is only 30 minutes left, slice the green onions and the sausages
7. Add the shrimp, the sausages and about ¾ of the green onions to your slow cooker
8. Cook your mixture for about ½ hour
9. Shred the slow cooked chicken with 2 forks
10. Ladle the gumbo into serving bowls; then sprinkle with the remaining green onions
11. Serve and enjoy your gumbo!

Nutrition Information

Calories: 312, Fat: 12g, Carbohydrates: 9g, Protein: 35g, Dietary Fiber 2g

Recipe 35: Shrimp Scampi

(Prep time: 6 Mins|Cook Time: 2 and ½ Hours| Servings: 3)

Ingredients

- ¼ Cup of chicken bone broth
- ½ Cup of water
- 2 Tablespoons of olive oil
- 2 Tablespoons of coconut oil
- 1 Tablespoon of minced garlic
- 2 Tablespoons of finely chopped parsley
- 1 Tablespoon of lemon juice
- 1 Pinch of salt
- 1 Pinch of pepper
- 1 Pound of raw peeled and deveined shrimp
- ½ Teaspoon of red pepper flakes

Instructions

1. Combine the broth with the water, the olive oil, the coconut oil, the garlic, the parsley, the salt and the pepper in a 2quart slow cooker
2. Add the shrimp to your slow cooker
3. Cover your slow cooker with a lid
4. Cook your ingredients for about 1 and ½ hours on High or for about 2 and ½ hours on Low
5. When the time is up; turn off your slow cooker
6. Serve and enjoy your meal!

Nutrition Information

Calories: 256, Fat: 14.7g, Carbohydrates: 2.7g, Protein: 23.5g, Dietary Fiber 0.2g

Recipe 36: Salmon chilli

(Prep time: 5 Mins|Cook Time: 2 Hours| Servings: 4-5)

Ingredients

- 4 Salmon fillets
- 2 Tablespoons of olive oil
- To prepare the marinade
- ¼ Cup of liquid aminos
- 1 Small handful of finely chopped baby spinach
- 1 Teaspoon of black pepper
- 2 Teaspoons of red pepper flakes
- To prepare the sweet chilli sauce topping:
- ¼ Cup of homemade chilli sauce

- 2 Teaspoon of extra virgin oil
- 1 Teaspoon of liquid aminos

Instructions

1. Preheat your slow cooker to Low and spray it with cooking spray
2. Make the marinade and mix it very well in a bowl
3. In a second medium bowl, make the topping of sweet chilli sauce and set it aside.
4. Place the salmon fillet in the marinade and coat it very well; then arrange the salmon fillet in the bottom of your slow cooker
5. Cover your slow cooker with a lid and cook on High for about 2 hours on High
6. When the time is up; turn off your slow cooker
7. Remove the salmon from the slow cooker and cover it with aluminium foil
8. Serve and enjoy your dish!

Nutrition Information

Calories: 198.8, Fat: 9.4g, Carbohydrates: 2.9g, Protein: 24.5g, Dietary Fiber 1.3g

Recipe 37: Shrimp zoodles

(Prep time: 5 Mins|Cook Time: 2 Hours| Servings: 4)

Ingredients

- 1 Tablespoon of coconut oil
- 2 Teaspoons of olive oil
- 1 Pound of peeled and deveined shrimp
- 1 Pinch of salt and 1 pinch of ground black pepper

- 3 Minced garlic cloves
- 1 Pinch of red pepper flakes
- 3 Medium zucchinis with the stems trimmed and Spiralized
- The zest and the juice of 1 lemon
- 2 Tablespoons of chopped fresh parsley

Instructions

1. Preheat your slow cooker to Low and spray it with cooking spray
2. Add the coconut oil to your slow cooker; then add the shrimp and season it with 1 pinch of salt and 1 pinch of pepper
3. Add in the garlic and the red pepper flakes and cover the slow cooker with its lid
4. Cook the shrimp for about 2 Hours on High
5. When the time is up, remove the lid and add in the zucchini noodles; the lemon juice and the zest and stir
6. Serve and enjoy your shrimp zoodles!

Nutrition Information

Calories: 225.7, Fat: 8.4g, Carbohydrates: 4g, Protein: 16g, Dietary Fiber 2.6g

Recipe 38: Fish cakes with avocado salsa

(Prep time: 10 Mins|Cook Time: 1 Hours| Servings: 7-8)

Ingredients

To make the salsa:
- 1 Diced mango
- 1 Chopped avocado

- ¼ Cubed red pepper
- 2 Tablespoons of diced red onion
- 2 Tablespoons of chopped cilantro
- The Juice of half a lime
- 1 Pinch of sea salt

Ingredients for the Thai fish cakes:

- 1 and ½ pounds of raw salmon with pin bones and the skin removed
- ½ Cup of canned coconut milk
- 2 Tablespoons of red Thai curry paste
- 2 Finely minced garlic cloves
- ½ Finely minced piece of 1 inch of ginger
- 1 Teaspoon of sriracha
- 1 Pasteurized large egg
- 2 Tablespoons of coconut oil

Instructions

- To make the salsa; combine all the ingredients in a bowl and stir very well; then set the mixture aside
- To make the Thai fish cakes:
- Pour the coconut milk in a large skillet; then add the curry paste, the garlic, the ginger and the sriracha and cook for about 8 minutes
- Break the salmon fish into small pieces with a spoon and cook for about 3 minutes
- Add in the pasteurized egg and mix again
- Preheat your slow cooker to Low and spray it with cooking spray
- Arrange the fish cakes in the bottom of your slow cooker and cover with a lid
- Cook for about 1 Hour on High
- When the time is up; turn off your slow cooker
- Serve and enjoy your fish cakes with salsa!

Nutrition Information

Calories: 303, Fat: 22g, Carbohydrates: 12g, Protein: 25.8g, Dietary Fiber 3.1g

Recipe 39: Slow cooked calamari with olives

(Prep time: 8 Mins|Cook Time: 6 Hours| Servings: 4)

Ingredients

- 1 and ½ pounds of cleaned squid
- 1 and ½ oz of smoked thinly sliced Spanish chorizo
- 1 Thinly sliced shallot
- 4 Thinly sliced garlic cloves
- 4 to 5 oil-packed anchovies
- 1 Thinly sliced red Fresno Chile or jalapeño
- 4 Tbsp of extra-virgin olive oil
- 1 Can of 28 of peeled tomatoes
- 1 Pinch of kosher salt
- 1 Pinch of freshly ground pepper
- 1 Cup of parsley leaves
- ½ Cup of mixed pitted green olives
- 2 Tablespoons of fresh lemon juice

Instructions

1. Preheat an oven to a temperature of 250°F.
2. Separate the squid bodies from the tentacles. Cut the bodies of the squid into thick rings and cut the tentacles into halves
3. Drain the squid and pat it dry; then cook the chorizo, the shallot, the garlic, the anchovies, the Chile, and about 2 Tbsp of oil in a large heavy pot over a medium high heat; then stir from time to time for about 5 minutes
4. Transfer the mixture to your slow cooker
5. Crush the tomatoes with your hands in a bowl; then add it to your slow cooker and stir
6. Season with 1 pinch of salt and 1 pinch of pepper
7. Cover your slow cooker with the lid and cook for about 3 hours on High or 6 hours on Low
8. Ladle you're the calamari dish in serving bowls and top it with parsley and olives

9. Serve and enjoy your dish!

Nutrition Information

Calories: 316, Fat: 14g, Carbohydrates: 10.8g, Protein: 32g, Dietary Fiber 2.9g

Recipe 40: Slow cooked Salmon with orange

(Prep time: 5 Mins|Cook Time: 1 and ½ Hours| Servings: 3)

Ingredients

- 2 large divided oranges
- 1 Cup of canned coconut milk
- 2 Tablespoons of coconut aminos
- 2 Tablespoons of finely minced ginger
- 1 Tablespoon of fish sauce
- 3 Finely sliced garlic cloves
- The juice of ½ Lime
- 4 to 5 Salmon fillets
- Chopped cilantro
- Orange zest
- 1 Pinch of black pepper

Instructions

1. Slice an orange; then place the zest and the juice of the orange in your slow cooker
2. Pour the coconut milk in your slow cooker with the coconut aminos, the ginger, the fish sauce, the garlic, and the lime juice to the slow cooker
3. Cover your slow cooker with a lid and cook on Low for about 1 hour
4. When the time is up; turn off your slow cooker

5. Lower the heat of your slow cooker and cook for about ½ hour on Low
6. Season with 1 pinch of salt and 1 pinch of pepper
7. Serve the salmon with black pepper and the orange sauce!

Nutrition Information

Calories: 335, Fat: 14g, Carbohydrates: 9.8g, Protein: 38g, Dietary Fiber 0.5g

Whole30 Slow Cooker Poultry Recipes

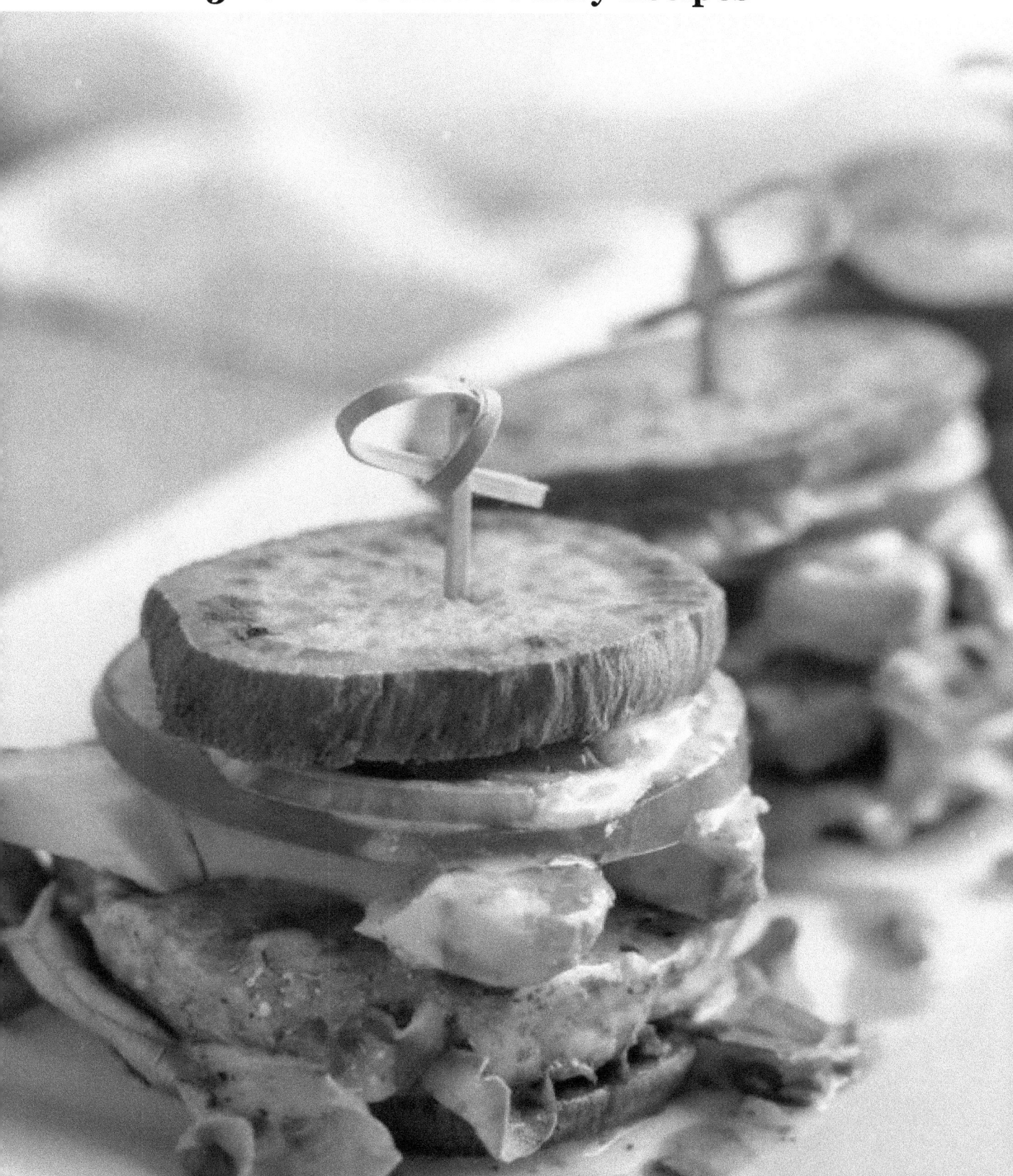

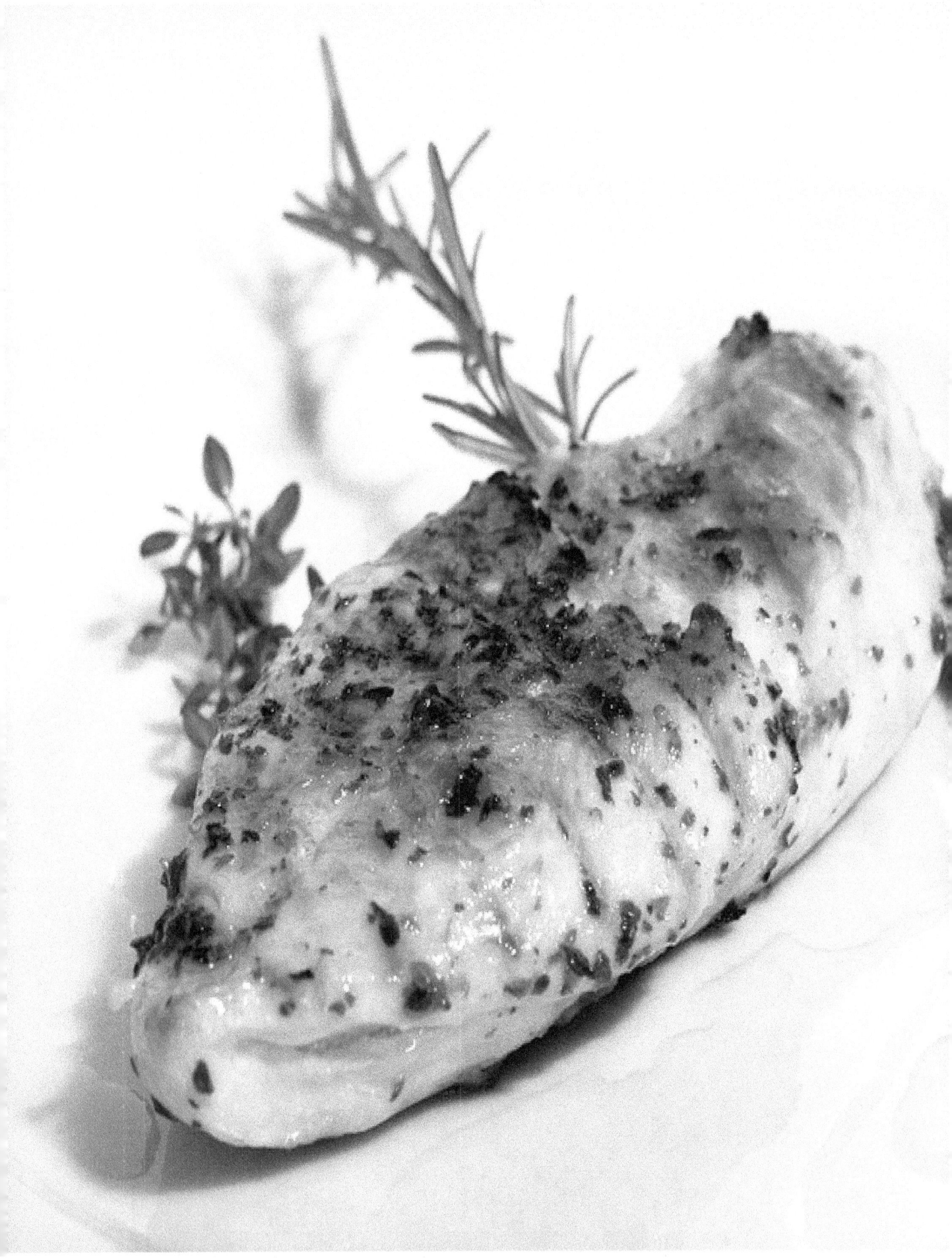

Recipe 41: Slow cooked chicken livers with mushrooms

(Prep time: 12 Mins|Cook Time: 5 Hours| Servings: 4)

Ingredients
- 1 Pound of chicken livers
- ½ Cup of arrowroot powder
- ½ Teaspoon of salt
- ¼ Teaspoon of pepper
- 8 Ounces of sliced mushrooms
- 4 Chopped green onions
- 1 Cup of chicken broth
- 1 Can of condensed golden mushroom soup
- ¼ Cup of vegetable broth

Instructions

1. Chop the chicken livers into small pieces
2. Combine the arrowroot powder with the salt and the pepper; then toss the chicken liver into the mixture
3. Add the livers, the green onions, and the sliced mushrooms to a large greased skillet and cook for about 4 minutes
4. Transfer the chicken liver to a slow cooker
5. Pour the chicken broth into your slow cooker; then add the vegetable soup and stir
6. Cover your slow cooker with a lid and cook on Low for about 3 to 5 hours
7. When the time is up; turn off your slow cooker
8. Serve and enjoy your chicken liver dish!
9.

Nutrition Information
Calories: 332, Fat: 18g, Carbohydrates: 13g, Protein: 28g, Dietary Fiber 2g

Recipe 42: Chicken Fajitas

(Prep time: 10 Mins|Cook Time: 6 Hours| Servings: 6)

Ingredients

- 1 Sliced orange bell pepper
- 1 Sliced into halves red bell pepper
- ½ Red sliced half red onion
- 3 to 4 large boneless chicken breasts
- 2 Tablespoons of taco seasoning

Instructions

1. Preheat your slow cooker to Low and spray it with cooking spray
2. Using a cutting board to make 5 horizontal slits in each of chicken breast, without cutting it all the way through
3. Rub the seasoning over the chicken breasts; then add more seasoning and coat the inside of the chicken slits
4. Stuff the chicken slits with the julienned bell peppers and the onions generously.
5. Arrange the stuffed chicken into the bottom of your slow cooker and close your slow cooker with a lid
6. Cook the chicken for about 3 hours on High or for about 6 hours on Low
7. When the time is up; turn off your slow cooker; remove the stuffed chicken and top it with cilantro and avocado
8. Serve and enjoy your meal!

Nutrition Information

Calories: 196, Fat: 10g, Carbohydrates: 8 g, Protein: 23g, Dietary Fiber 0.3g

Recipe 43: Artichoke Chicken casserole

(Prep time: 7 Mins|Cook Time: 3 and ½ Hours| Servings: 3-4)

Ingredients

- 2 Pounds of boneless and skinless chicken breasts
- ¾ Teaspoon of kosher salt
- 1/2 Teaspoon of freshly ground black pepper
- 1 and ½ cups of thawed or drained frozen artichoke hearts
- 2 Smashed garlic cloves
- 1 Medium halved and thinly sliced shallot
- 1 Cut into wedges medium lemon
- ½ Cup of low-sodium chicken broth
- ½ cup of chicken broth
- 3 Ounces of baby spinach
- Finely chopped fresh parsley leaves

Instructions

1. Start by seasoning the chicken breasts with 1 pinch of salt and 1 pinch of pepper
2. Arrange the chicken in the bottom of a 6-quart or larger slow cooker into 1 layer
3. Slice the hearts of artichoke into halves; then add it to your slow cooker
4. Scatter the shallot, the garlic and the lemon wedges over the artichokes and the chicken
5. Pour the chicken broth in your slow cooker
6. Cover your slow cooker with a lid and cook on Low for about 3 and ½ hours
7. When the time is up; transfer the slow cooked chicken to a serving dish.

8. Add the spinach to your slow cooker and toss it with the lemon and artichoke
9. Transfer your slow cooked chicken and artichokes into a serving dish
10. Top with parsley; then serve and enjoy your dish!

Nutrition Information

Calories: 223.2, Fat: 5.7g, Carbohydrates: 11.2 g, Protein: 27.4g, Dietary Fiber 3.2g

Recipe 44: Chicken skewers

(Prep time: 5 Mins|Cook Time: 2 Hours| Servings: 5)

Ingredients

- 1 Pound of ground chicken
- 1 Small chopped onion
- 2 Minced garlic cloves
- 1 Tablespoon of parsley
- 2 Teaspoons of coriander
- 1 Teaspoon of cumin
- ½ Teaspoon of salt
- ½ Teaspoon of pepper
- ¼ Teaspoon of nutmeg
- ¼ Teaspoon of mint
- ¼ Teaspoon of paprika

Instructions

1. Preheat your slow cooker to Low and line it with a baking paper

2. Add all the ingredients to a medium bowl.
3. Mix your ingredients together until the spices and the onion until it becomes very well blended
4. Shape the meat with your hands and evenly place it over skewers
5. Spray the baking paper in the slow cooker with cooking spray
6. Place the skewers in your slow cooker and cover it with a lid
7. Cook on high for about 2 hours or on Low for about 4 hours
8. When the time is up; turn off your slow cooker
9. Serve and enjoy your skewers!

Nutrition Information

Calories: 145, Fat: 3.5g, Carbohydrates: 1.8 g, Protein: 26g, Dietary Fiber 0.4g

Recipe 45: Chicken with pineapple

(Prep time: 10Mins|Cook Time: 1 Hour| Servings: 3)

Ingredients

- 3 Pounds of boneless and skinless chicken thighs
- 1 and ½ cups of pineapple juice
- 2 Inches of roughly chopped ginger piece
- 3 Tablespoons of coconut aminos
- ⅓ Cup of chopped pitted dates
- 2 Tablespoons of apple cider vinegar
- 1 Teaspoon of salt
- 1 Pinch of pepper
- 2 Tablespoons of arrowroot
- 3 Minced garlic cloves
- 1 Chopped red pepper
- 3 Diced green onions

- 1 Cup of chopped fresh pineapple

Instructions

1. Place the chicken in the bottom of your slow cooker.
2. Prepare the sauce by combining the pineapple juice, the ginger, the coconut aminos, the dates, the salt and the pepper and blend it with a blender
3. Pour the mixture over the chicken and add in the minced garlic.
4. Cover your slow cooker with a lid and cook on Low for about 3 hours
5. Mix the arrowroot into about ¼ cup of water and combine it very well
6. Pour the arrowroot slurry over the chicken in your slow cooker and cook on Low for about 1 hour
7. When the time is up; turn off your slow cooker
8. Ladle your chicken dish in serving plate and top with chopped green onions and crushed red bell pepper
9. Serve and enjoy!

Nutrition Information

Calories: 222, Fat: 7.2g, Carbohydrates: 11g, Protein: 27g, Dietary Fiber 0.3g

Recipe 46: Slow cooked Cornish hens with sweet potatoes and green beans

(Prep time: 7 Mins|Cook Time: 4 Hours| Servings: 3)

Ingredients

- 2 to 3 Cornish hens
- 1 Pound of peeled and diced sweet potatoes
- 1 Sliced small onion
- 1 Pound of green beans
- To make the spice blend:

- 1 Teaspoon of garlic powder
- 1 Teaspoon of paprika
- 1 Teaspoon of salt
- ½ Teaspoon of onion powder
- ½ Teaspoon of oregano
- ½ Teaspoon of thyme
- ½ Teaspoon of cayenne
- ½ Teaspoon of pepper

Instructions

1. Add the sweet potatoes, the green beans, and the onion to the bottom of your slow cooker.
2. Place the Cornish Hens right over the top of your ingredients
3. Sprinkle the spice blend over your ingredients in your slow cooker
4. Cover your slow cooker with a lid and cook on High for about 3 to 4 hours on High or on Low for about 5 to 6 hours
5. When the time is up; turn off your slow cooker
6. Serve and enjoy your meal!

Nutrition Information

Calories: 207.6, Fat: 10.9g, Carbohydrates: 2.4 g, Protein: 24.3g, Dietary Fiber 0.8g

Recipe 47: Garlicky chicken drumsticks

(Prep time: 4 Mins|Cook Time: 4 Hours| Servings: 6)

Ingredients

- 2 Pounds of chicken drumsticks
- 4 Teaspoons of chopped garlic

- 2 Sprigs of rosemary
- 3 Tablespoons of olive oil
- ½ Cup of chicken stock

Instructions

1. Preheat your slow cooker to Low and spray it with cooking spray
2. Combine the chicken drumsticks with the garlic, the rosemary and the olive oil
3. Shake your ingredients very well.
4. Add the chicken mixture to your slow cooker; then pour in the chicken stock
5. Cook the chicken drumsticks for about 4 hour on High
6. Transfer the chicken to a pan and broil the chicken for about 3 minutes per each side
7. Garnish with fresh herb; then serve and enjoy your dish!

Nutrition Information

Calories: 248, Fat: 15.4g, Carbohydrates: 8.3 g, Protein: 29.3g, Dietary Fiber 0.6g

Recipe 48: Chicken teriyaki

(Prep time: 5 Mins|Cook Time: 4-5 Hours| Servings: 3)

Ingredients

- 2 Pounds of boneless or bone-in skinless chicken thighs
- ½ Cup of coconut aminos
- 1 Pinch of salt
- 1 Tablespoon of grated fresh ginger

- 2 Minced garlic cloves
- 1 Pinch of black pepper

Instructions

1. Place the chicken in your slow cooker.
2. Mix the coconut aminos, the fresh ginger and the garlic cloves.
3. Pour the prepared sauce over the chicken meat and place the mixture in the bottom of a greased slow cooker
4. Cover your slow cooker with a lid and cook on Low for about 4 to 5 hours on Low.
5. Remove the chicken from your slow cooker and adjust the seasoning of salt and pepper
6. Serve and enjoy your meal!

Nutrition Information

Calories: 270, Fat: 6g, Carbohydrates: 14g, Protein: 16g, Dietary Fiber 3.7g

Recipe 49: Chicken with Garlic and Citrus

(Prep time: 5 Mins|Cook Time: 5 Hours| Servings: 4)

Ingredients

- 2 Pounds of chicken
- 1 Sliced onion
- 1 Sliced lemon
- To make the sauce:
- 7 Minced garlic cloves
- ¼ Cup of lime juice
- ¼ Cup of orange juice

- 2 Tablespoons of evoo
- 1 Teaspoon of salt
- 1 Teaspoon of oregano
- ¼ Teaspoon of cumin

Instructions

1. Add the sliced onion to the bottom of your slow cooker.
2. Add the chicken on top of the onion
3. In a bowl, mix all the ingredients together
4. Pour the sauce on top of your ingredients and mix
5. Top with the sliced lemon
6. Cover your slow cooker with a lid
7. Cook on High for about 2 to 3 hours or on Low for about 4 to 5 hours
8. When the time is up; turn off your slow cooker
9. Serve and enjoy your meal!

Nutrition Information

Calories: 185, Fat: 9.7g, Carbohydrates: 12.1 g, Protein: 13.8g, Dietary Fiber 1.4g

Recipe 50: Chicken patties

(Prep time: 8 Mins|Cook Time: 3 Hours| Servings: 7-8)

Ingredients

- 1 Pound of ground chicken
- 3 Chopped green onions
- ¼ Cup of Red Hot sauce
- 2 tablespoons of vegan mayonnaise
- ½ Teaspoon of salt
- 1 Pasteurized egg

Instructions

1. Preheat your slow cooker to Low and spray it with cooking spray
2. Combine the ground chicken with the green onions, the hot sauce, the pasteurized egg, the vegan mayonnaise and the salt in a large bowl
3. Make small balls from the chicken mixture; then arrange the balls in the bottom of your slow cooker and cover it with its lid
4. Cook the chicken balls for about 3 Hours on High
5. Remove the chicken balls from the slow cooker and drizzle with hot sauce; then top with green onions
6. Serve and enjoy your dish!

Nutrition Information

Calories: 160, Fat: 8g, Carbohydrates: 12.3g, Protein: 14g, Dietary Fiber 0.5g

Whole30 Slow Cooker Soup and stew Recipes

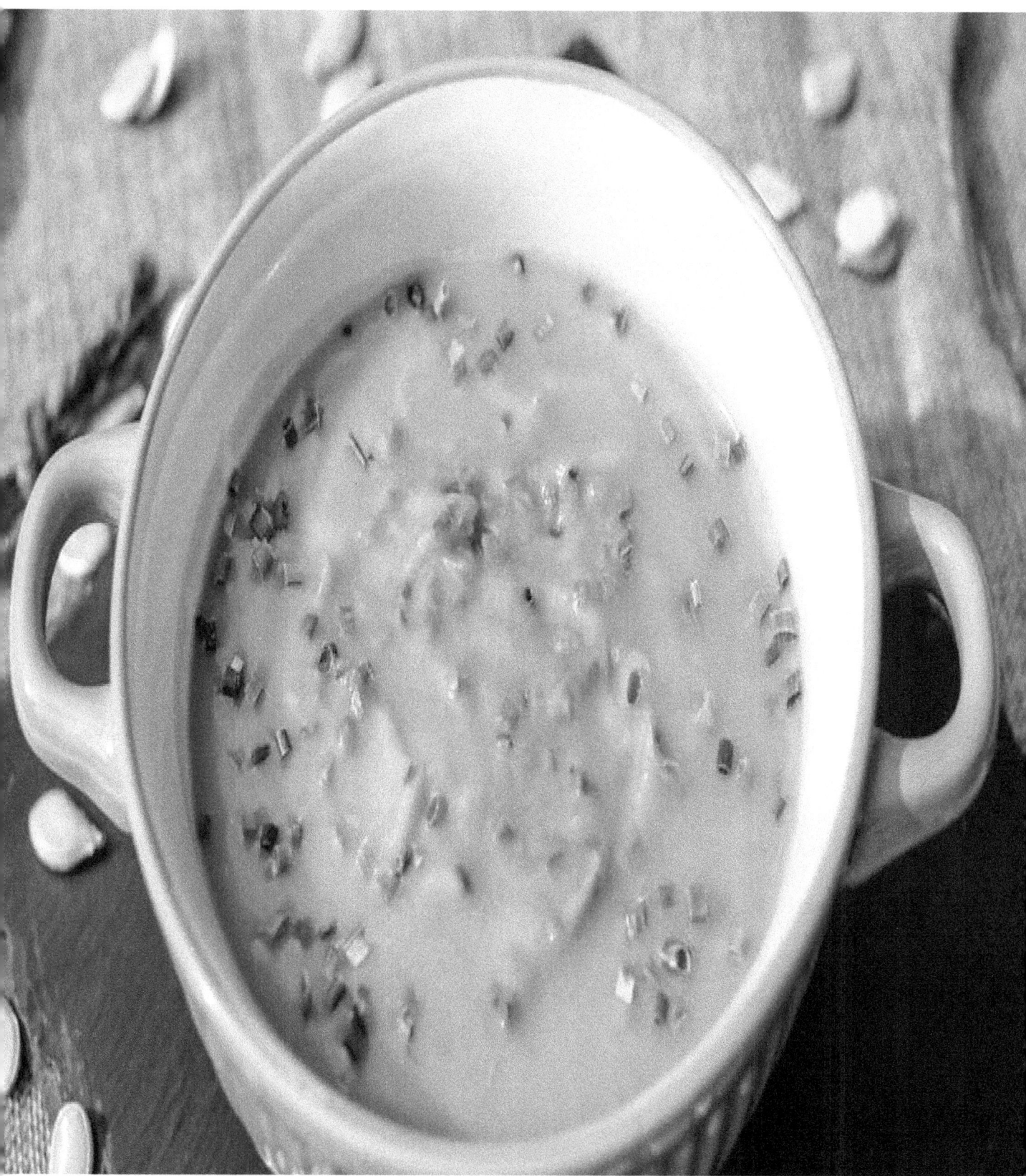

Recipe 51: Beef and cabbage stew

(Prep time: 5 Mins|Cook Time: 8 Hours| Servings: 4)

Ingredients

- 1 Pound of ground beef
- 4 Cups of roughly chopped red and green cabbage
- 2 to 3 Diced carrots
- 1 Diced onion
- 2 Cups of chopped fresh tomatoes
- 4 garlic cloves, minced
- 2 Cups of tomato sauce
- 4 and ½ cups of beef or chicken stock
- 1 Teaspoon of paprika
- 1 Teaspoon of dried oregano
- ½ Teaspoon of dried basil
- 1 Tablespoon of coconut oil
- 1 Pinch of salt
- 1 Pinch of freshly ground black pepper

Instructions

1. Melt the coconut oil in a large skillet over a medium high heat
2. Add the onion and the garlic and cook for about 2 to 3 minutes
3. Add in the beef and brown it for about 4 minutes
4. Transfer your ingredients to the slow cooker; then season with 1 pinch of salt and 1 pinch of pepper
5. Add the beef and the rest of the ingredients to your slow cooker and cover with the lid
6. Cook your stew for about 6 to 8 hours on Low or on high for about 4 to 5 hours
7. Serve and enjoy your slow cooked stew!

Nutrition Information

Calories: 237, Fat: 3.52g, Carbohydrates: 10 g, Protein: 17.4g, Dietary Fiber 2.7g

Recipe 52: Sweet potato soup

(Prep time: 5 Mins|Cook Time: 5 Hours| Servings: 4)

Ingredients
- 2 Tablespoons of olive oil
- 1 Pound of ground turkey
- 1 Medium chopped white onion
- 3 Minced garlic cloves
- 2 large skinned and chopped sweet potatoes
- 10 Oz of sliced mushrooms
- 5 Cups of chicken broth
- 2 Tablespoons of apple cider vinegar
- 1 Tablespoon of dried basil
- 1 Teaspoon of sea salt
- ½ Teaspoon of fresh ground pepper
- 3 Cups of roughly chopped kale
- 2 Tablespoons of freshly chopped thyme

Instructions
1. Heat a large and heavy skillet to a medium high heat; then coat the skillet with oil
2. Add the sausage and cook for about 5 minutes
3. Add in the onion and the garlic; then cook for about 3 minutes
4. Transfer the sausage mixture to your slow cooker; then add in the sweet potatoes, the mushrooms, the chicken broth, the vinegar, the basil, the salt, and the pepper.
5. Cover your slow cooker with a lid and cook on Low for about 4 hours
6. Add the kale and stir your soup; then cook for about 15 additional minutes
7. Serve and enjoy your soup with chopped fresh thyme!

Nutrition Information
Calories: 190.6, Fat: 6g, Carbohydrates: 11 g, Protein: 12.7g, Dietary Fiber 3.1g

Recipe 53: Liver stew

(Prep time: 4 Mins|Cook Time: 2 Hours| Servings: 3)

Ingredients

- 1 and ½ pounds of lamb's liver
- 2 Tablespoons of oil
- 8 Oz of sliced onion
- 14 Oz of chopped tomatoes
- 3 Tablespoons of cold water
- 1 Tablespoon of lamb seasoning

Instructions

1. Pre-heat your slow cooker to Low and spray it with cooking spray
2. Slice the liver and pat it dry with paper towels
3. Add the liver to the bottom of your slow cooker; then add the onion
4. Add the tomatoes and the water
5. Season with 1 pinch of salt and 1 pinch of pepper
6. Cover with a lid and cook for about 2 hours on High
7. When the time is up, turn off your slow cooker
8. Serve and enjoy your stew!

Nutrition Information

Calories: 138, Fat: 2.92g, Carbohydrates: 11 g, Protein: 12.6g, Dietary Fiber 2.1g

Recipe 54: Chicken and mushroom soup

(Prep time: 8 Mins|Cook Time: 4 Hours| Servings: 3)

Ingredients
- ½ Sliced sweet Yellow Onion
- 1 Tablespoon of Olive Oil
- 1 Pound of Boneless Skinless Chicken Tenders
- 25 Oz of sliced Crimini Mushrooms
- 6 Chopped Garlic Cloves
- 4 Cups of Mushroom or Chicken Broth
- ¼ Teaspoon of Salt
- ¼ Teaspoon of Pepper
- ¼ Teaspoon of Garlic Powder
- ¼ Teaspoon of Onion Powder
- 1/8 Teaspoon of Dried Thyme

Instructions
1. Sauté the onions in a large skillet over a medium high heat for about 7 minutes
2. Spray your slow cooker with cooking spray and add in the mushrooms, the garlic and the onion
3. Oil your slow cooker and arrange the chicken in the bottom in 1 layer
4. Pour the broth over the chicken in your slow cooker
5. Season with 1 pinch of salt and 1 pinch of pepper
6. Add the garlic powder, the onion powder and the thyme
7. Cover your slow cooker with a lid and cook on High for about 3 to 4 hours
8. When the time is up; turn off your slow cooker; then shred the chicken
9. Serve and enjoy your soup in bowls that you can top with parsley!

Nutrition Information
Calories: 112.5, Fat: 2.7g, Carbohydrates: 12.5 g, Protein: 11.9g, Dietary Fiber 2.3g

Recipe 55: Cauliflower soup

(Prep time: 8 Mins|Cook Time: 6 Hours| Servings: 3)

Ingredients

- 1 Medium cored and chopped into small pieces head of cauliflower
- 1 Medium peeled and chopped white sweet potato
- 2 Tablespoons of avocado oil
- 1 Tablespoon of minced garlic
- 1 Medium diced yellow onion
- 3 Cups of chicken broth
- ½ Cup of water
- 1 Cup of coconut milk
- 1 and ½ teaspoons of truffle salt
- ½ Teaspoon of turmeric
- ½ Teaspoon of ground black pepper
- Finely chopped scallions
- Cooled Pancetta

Instructions

1. Place all your ingredients in your slow cooker except for the coconut milk
2. Cover your slow cooker with a lid and cook on Low for about 6 hours
3. When the time is up; turn off your slow cooker; then add the coconut milk and blend your ingredients until it becomes smooth
4. Season with 1 pinch of salt and 1 pinch of pepper
5. Ladle the soup in serving bowls and garnish with chopped scallions
6. Serve and enjoy your soup!

Nutrition Information
Calories: 114, Fat: 5.2g, Carbohydrates: 13 g, Protein: 5g, Dietary Fiber 2.3g

Whole30 Slow cooker appetizer and snack Recipes

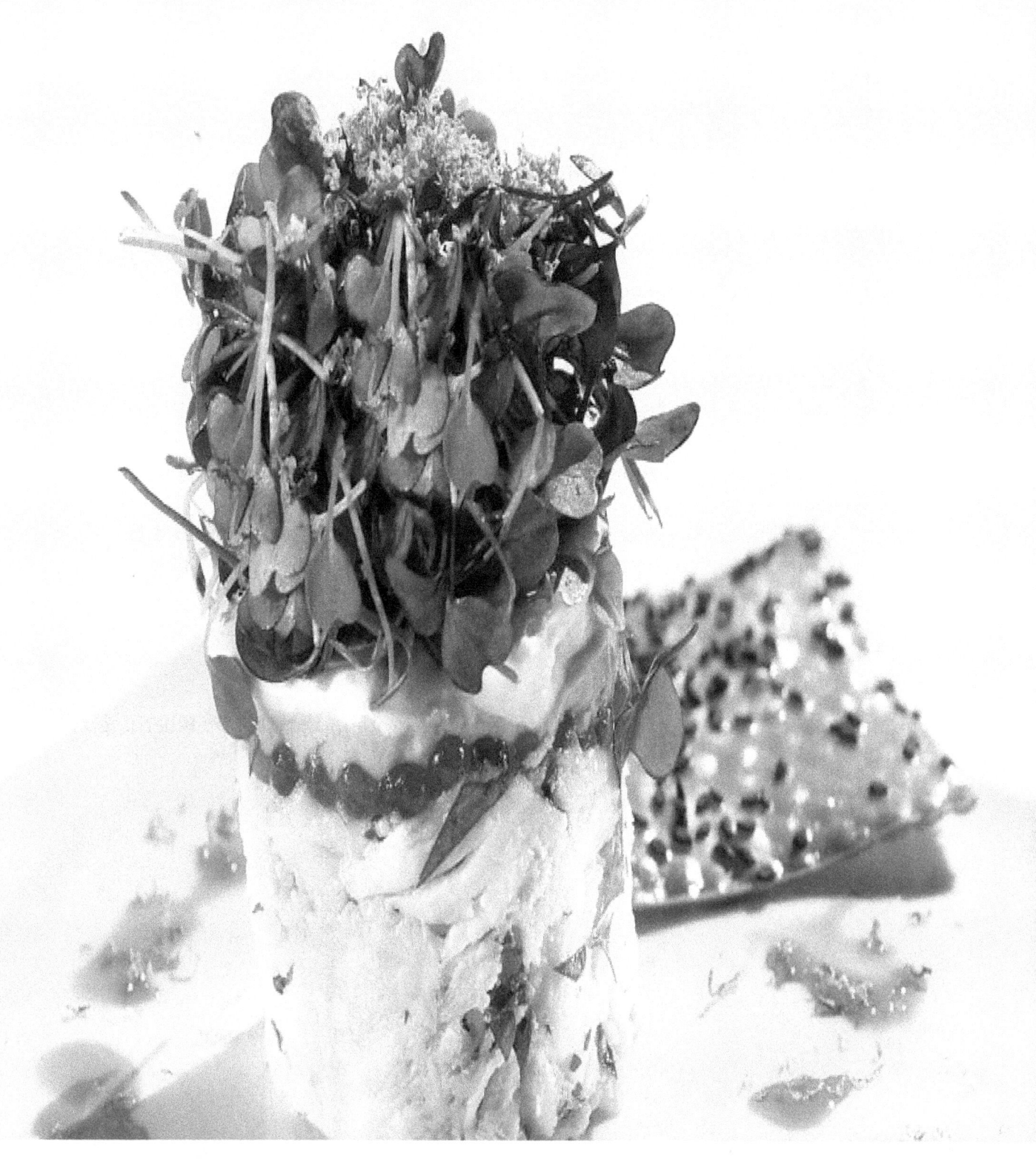

Recipe 56: Stuffed mushrooms

(Prep time: 5 Mins|Cook Time: 3 Hours| Servings: 7-8)

Ingredients

- 12 Wiped with the stem removed button mushrooms
- ½ Pound of Italian sausage
- 1 Pasteurized egg white
- ¼ Cup of sugar-free marinara sauce

Instructions

1. Preheat your slow cooker to Low and spray it with cooking spray
2. Remove the stems of your slow cooker and wipe it with a clean paper towel
3. Place the Italian sausage into a bowl and mix it with the pasteurized egg
4. Use your hands to combine the meat
5. Make small balls from the mixture; then stuff the mushrooms with the mixtures
6. Arrange the mushrooms in the bottom of your slow cooker and pour the sauce
7. Cover the slow cooker with the lid and cook on High for about 1 and ½ hours on High or on Low for about 3 hours
8. When the time is up; turn off your slow cooker
9. Serve and enjoy your appetizer!

Nutrition Information

Calories: 172.5, Fat: 10.4g, Carbohydrates: 4.6 g, Protein: 15g, Dietary Fiber 1.3g

Recipe 57: Zucchini rolls

(Prep time: 10 Mins|Cook Time: 2 Hours| Servings: 11-12)

Ingredients

- 2 Sliced zucchinis with the ends removed
- 4 to 5 Italian sausages
- ½ Cup of walnuts
- 1 Cup of fresh basil
- 1/3 Cup of olive oil
- The juice of 1 lemon
- 1 Minced garlic clove
- 1Pinch of salt and 1 pinch of pepper
- 1 Pinch of garlic powder
- 3 Tablespoons of olive oil

Instructions

1. Slice the zucchini; then place it in a bowl with about 3 tablespoons of olive oil
2. Add 1 pinch of salt and 1 pinch of pepper
3. Add 1 pinch of garlic powder; then coat the zucchini with the mixture of oil
4. Grill the zucchini for about 3 minutes
5. Place the sausages into the middle of each of the zucchini slices; then roll the zucchinis over the sausages
6. Carefully arrange the rolled zucchinis into the bottom of your slow cooker and cover the slow cooker with the lid
7. Cook on Low for about 2 hours
8. In the meantime, make the pesto by adding the walnuts, the garlic clove, and the basil a food processor and puree it for a few seconds; then start gradually adding the olive oil
9. Add the lemon juice, the salt and the pepper; then add more basil, lemon and pepper
10. When the timer of your slow cooker is up; turn it off

11. Slice the zucchini rolls into halves
12. Serve and enjoy your snack!

Nutrition Information

Calories: 90.9, Fat: 5g, Carbohydrates: 1.5 g, Protein: 4.3g, Dietary Fiber 0.2g

Recipe 58: Artichoke and cashews dip

(Prep time: 7 Mins|Cook Time: 4 Hours| Servings: 3)

Ingredients

- 1 Cup of raw cashews
- 1 Cup of almond milk
- 2 Roughly chopped garlic cloves
- 1 Teaspoon of kosher salt
- 2 Tablespoons of fresh lemon juice
- 2 Teaspoons of Dijon mustard
- 1 Bag of 8 oz of frozen defrosted and squeezed spinach
- 2 Cans of 4 oz of drained, rinsed and roughly chopped artichoke hearts
- 1 Can of 8 oz of diced drained and rinsed water chestnuts
- 2 Tablespoons of nutritional yeast
- 3 Tablespoons of avocado vegan mayonnaise
- 1 Pinch of freshly ground pepper

Instructions

1. Start by processing the cashews with a blender

2. Add the almond milk, the garlic, the salt, the lemon juice and the mustard; then blend on High until you obtain a smooth mixture
3. Pour the mixture in a 4-quart slow cooker
4. Add the artichoke hearts, the water chestnuts and the nutritional yeast and stir
5. Cover your slow cooker with the lid and cook on Low for about 3 to 4 hours on Low or 2 hours on High
6. Uncover your slow cooker and stir in the mayonnaise
7. Adjust the seasoning with salt and pepper
8. Serve and enjoy your dip!

Nutrition Information

Calories: 173.5, Fat: 5.7g, Carbohydrates: 12.4 g, Protein: 16.5g, Dietary Fiber 2.6g

Recipe 59: Mashed sweet potatoes

(Prep time: 6 Mins|Cook Time: 3and ½ Hours| Servings: 3)

Ingredients

- 2 Pounds of peeled and cubed sweet potatoes
- 1 Cup of water
- ¼ Cup of clarified ghee
- 4 Finely chopped garlic cloves
- ½ Teaspoon of sea salt
- ½ Cup of Primal Kitchen Ranch Dressing
- ¼ Cup of nutritional yeast
- ¼ Cup of chopped chives

Instructions

1. Chop the potatoes into cubes of 1 and ½ inches each
2. Add the ghee, the garlic and the salt to the potatoes
3. Place your ingredients in your slow cooker.
4. Add the ghee, the liquid, the garlic and the salt.
5. Place the lid on your slow cooker and set the heat to High
6. Cook on High for about 3 and ½ hours
7. Mash the sweet potatoes with a masher or an immersion blender
8. Add the ranch dressing and the chives and stir again
9. Serve and enjoy your nutritious appetizer!

Nutrition Information

Calories: 100, Fat: 8g, Carbohydrates: 5 g, Protein: 4g, Dietary Fiber 2g

Recipe 60: Liver pate

(Prep time: 5 Mins|Cook Time: 1 and ½ Hours| Servings: 4)

Ingredients

- 1 Small, minced onion
- 4 Minced garlic cloves
- 1 Pound of grass-fed beef liver
- 2 Tablespoons of minced fresh
- 2 Tablespoons of minced fresh thyme
- ½ Cup of melted coconut oil
- ½ Teaspoon of sea salt
- Sliced fresh carrots and cucumber

Instructions

1. Grease a large skillet over a medium high heat; then brown the liver for about 2 minutes
2. Transfer the liver meat to a slow cooker and add the garlic to it
3. Add the herbs and 1 cup of water; then season with 1 pinch of salt and 1 pinch of pepper
4. Cover your slow cooker with a lid and cook for about 1 and ½ hours on High
5. When the time is up, turn off your slow cooker
6. Remove the liver from the slow cooker and transfer the ingredients to a food processor or a blender with the coconut oil and the sea salt and blend for about 2 minutes or until the ingredients become smooth
7. Serve the liver pate in a serving dish and top it with chopped fresh herbs, carrot slices and cucumber slices
8. Enjoy!

Nutrition Information

Calories: 85.4, Fat: 8g, Carbohydrates: 2.1 g, Protein: 5.6g, Dietary Fiber 0.3g

Whole30 Slow Cooker Salad Recipes

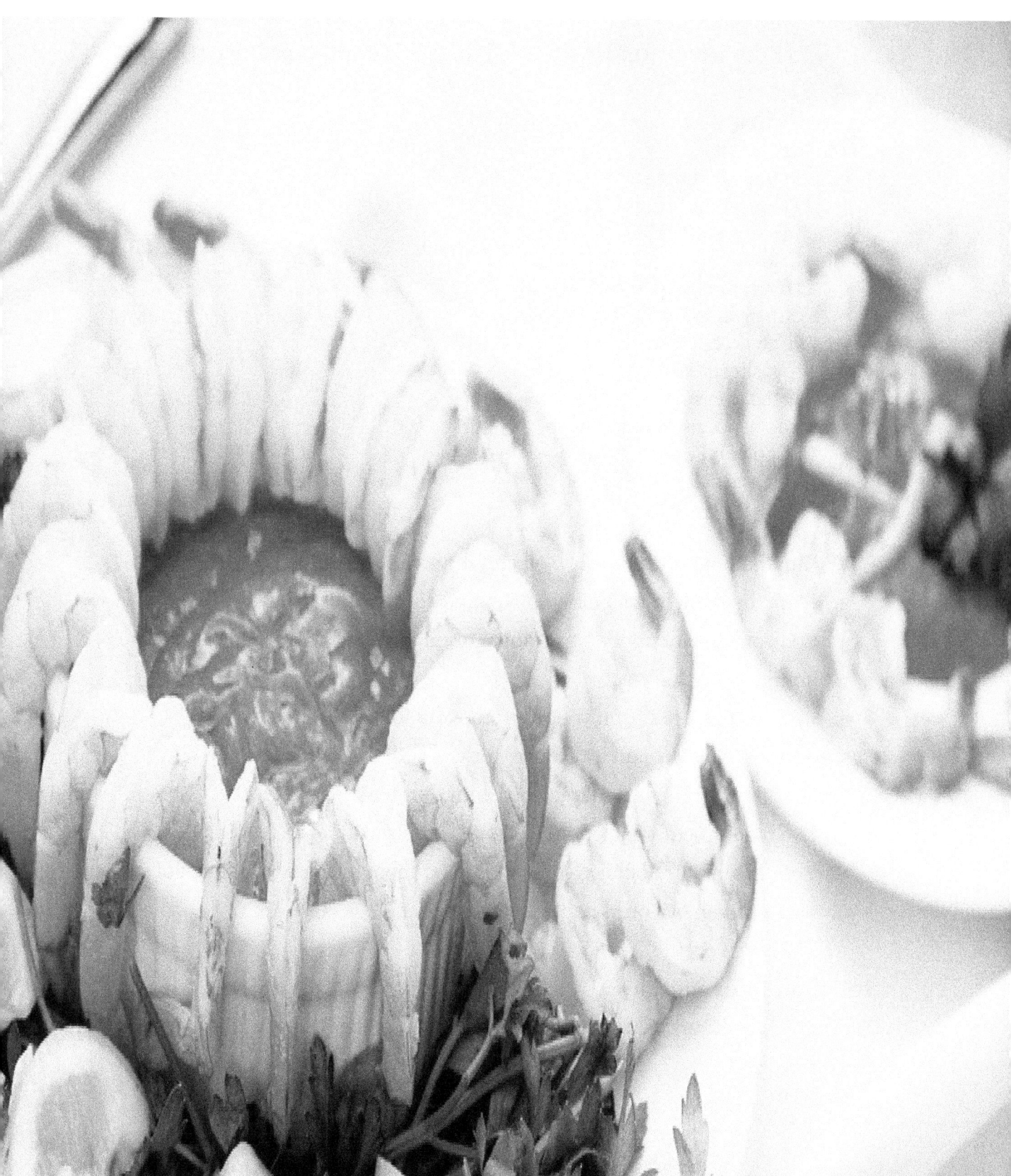

Recipe 61: Beef salad

(Prep time: 10 Mins|Cook Time: 8 Hours| Servings: 3)

Ingredients
For the beef steak:
- 2 Pounds of skirt steak
- 2 Tablespoons of olive oil
- 1 Tablespoon of steak seasoning

For the salad:
- 2 Heads of chopped romaine hearts
- 1 Cup of sliced grape tomatoes
- 1 large sliced avocado
- 4 to 5 sliced baby sweet peppers
- For the dressing:
- 2 Tablespoons of lime juice
- ¼ Cup of cilantro
- 1 Pinch of salt

Instructions
1. Rub the steak with the olive oil and the steak seasoning
2. Place the steak in your slow cooker and cover with the lid
3. Cook on Low for about 7 to 8 hours or on High for about 3 and ½ to 4 hours
4. Remove the steak from your slow cooker and set it aside to cool
5. Slice the steak or pull it with two forks
6. Toss the veggies into a large bowl with the steak
7. In a food processor; blend the cilantro with the lime juice
8. Pour the mixture of juices over the steak; then season with 1 pinch of salt
9. Serve and enjoy your salad!

Nutrition Information
Calories: 322, Fat: 21g, Carbohydrates: 12g, Protein: 36g, Dietary Fiber 3g

Recipe 62: Sweet potato Salad

(Prep time: 6 Mins|Cook Time: 5 Hours| Servings: 3-4)

Ingredients
- 4 Medium, peeled and chopped sweet potatoes into cubes of ½ inch each
- 1 Tablespoon of avocado oil
- ½ Teaspoon of sea salt divided
- ½ Cup of chipotle lime vegan mayonnaise
- 1 Juiced lime
- 1 Cup of diced celery
- ¼ Cup of diced red pepper
- ¼ Cup of diced red onion
- ¼ Cup of chopped fresh cilantro

Instructions
1. Preheat your slow cooker to Low and spray it with cooking spray
2. Add in the sweet potatoes and drizzle with olive oil
3. Sprinkle with 1 pinch of salt and 1 pinch of pepper and cover the slow cooker with a lid
4. Cook on Low for about 5 hours or on High for about 2 and ½ hours
5. When the time is up; turn off your slow cooker
6. Whisk the chipotle lime vegan mayo, the lime juice, and the remaining sea salt all together into a large bowl
7. Add in the red onion, the red pepper and the celery
8. When the time is up; turn off your slow cooker and toss the sweet potatoes in a large bowl with the mayonnaise mixture.
9. Fold in the cilantro and gently mix
10. Serve and enjoy your salad!

Nutrition Information
Calories: 181.1, Fat: 4g, Carbohydrates: 11.6g, Protein: 28.3g, Dietary Fiber 0.7g

Recipe 63: Turkey salad

(Prep time: 5 Mins|Cook Time: 8 Hours| Servings: 3)

Ingredients

- 1 Pound of ground turkey
- ¼ Cup of chopped onion
- 2 tablespoons of diced jalapeno
- 1 package of taco seasoning
- 1 package of ranch dressing
- 2 tablespoons of water
- 1 head of cleaned and chopped romaine lettuce

Optional toppings:
- Chopped grape tomatoes
- Sliced avocados

Instructions

- Place the raw ground turkey in your slow cooker and break it up with a spatula
- Add the onions, the jalapenos, the taco seasoning, the ranch dressing and the water
- Stir your ingredients very well
- Cover your slow cooker with the lid and cook on Low for about 6 to 8 hours on Low or for about 3 to 4 hours on High
- When the time is up; turn off your slow cooker
- Serve your salad with lettuce and avocado slices
- Serve and enjoy your salad!

Nutrition Information

Calories: 222, Fat: 10.6g, Carbohydrates: 12g, Protein: 14.5g, Dietary Fiber 1g

Recipe 64: Lamb salad

(Prep time: 10 Mins|Cook Time: 6Hours| Servings: 3-4)

Ingredients
- 2 Minced garlic cloves
- The zest of 1 lemon
- 4 Chopped oregano sprigs
- 1 tbsp of extra virgin olive oil
- 2 Pounds of trimmed of fat lamb shoulder
- 1 Cup of chicken stock
- ½ Pound of chopped pumpkin
- 2 Tablespoons of olive oil
- ½ Pound of halved cherry tomato
- 1 Cup of baby spinach
- 1 Tablespoon of balsamic vinegar
- 2 Teaspoons of olive oil

Instructions
1. Preheat your slow cooker to Low
2. Combine the garlic, the lemon zest and the juice with the oregano and the olive oil in a large bowl.
3. Add the lamb to your slow cooker and season it with 1 pinch of salt and 1 pinch of pepper
4. Pour 1 cup of stock over the mixture and Put the marinade over the lamb and cover the slow cooker with the lid
5. Cook on High for about 3 hours or on Low for about 6 hours
6. When the time is up, turn off your slow cooker and roast the chopped pumpkin in a greased baking tray in a preheated oven
7. Remove the lamb from the slow cooker and the pumpkin from the oven
8. Combine the tomatoes with the pumpkin, the spinach, the vinegar and the olive oil; then add the lamb
9. Drizzle with the juices and season with 1 pinch of salt
10. Serve and enjoy your salad!

Nutrition Information
Calories: 312, Fat: 17.3g, Carbohydrates: 9g, Protein: 18.5g, Dietary Fiber 0.4g

Recipe 65: Cauliflower salad

(Prep time: 5 Mins|Cook Time: 1 Hour| Servings: 3)

Ingredients
- 1 and ½ pounds of trimmed and chopped cauliflower
- ¾ Cup of chopped bottled roasted red bell peppers
- ½ Cup of thinly sliced red onion
- ½ Cup of coarsely chopped fresh flat-leaf parsley
- ½ Cup of coarsely chopped green olives
- ¼ Teaspoon of crushed red pepper
- 1 Sliced celery rib
- 2 Tablespoons of extra-virgin olive oil
- 1 Tablespoon of fresh lemon juice
- 1 Tablespoon of apple vinegar
- ½ Teaspoon of black pepper
- 1/8 Teaspoon of sea salt
- Celery leaves

Instructions
1. Toss the cauliflower florets in your slow cooker and pour in 1 cup of water
2. Sprinkle 1 pinch of salt
3. Lock the slow cooker with a lid and cook on High for about 1 hour
4. When the time is up, turn off your slow cooker
5. Transfer the cauliflower to a bowl and add in the bell peppers, the red onion, the parsley, the chopped olives, the crushed and red pepper
6. Add the celery and combine very well
7. Mix the oil with the juice, the vinegar, the black pepper, and the salt; then stir and pour the dressing over your vegetables
8. Serve and enjoy your salad!

Nutrition Information
Calories: 234, Fat: 11g, Carbohydrates: 10g, Protein: 5.6g, Dietary Fiber 2.8g

Recipe 66: Chicken Salad

(Prep time: 8 Mins|Cook Time: 2 and ½ Hours| Servings: 3)

Ingredients

For the slow Cooker Chicken:
- 1 and ¾ pounds of chicken breast
- 1 Tablespoon of minced garlic
- ½ Teaspoon of paprika
- ¼ Teaspoon of chilli powder
- 1 and ½ cups of sugar-free chicken broth

For the Chipotle Lime Chicken Salad:
- 2 Cups of shredded chicken
- 1/3 cup of Whole30 Mayonnaise
- 1 Handful of cilantro

For the avocado Curry Chicken Salad:
- 2 Cups of shredded chicken
- ½ Medium, pitted and fleshed avocado
- 1 to 2 teaspoons of curry powder
- 1/4 Teaspoon of pink salt

Instructions

1. Cut any excess of fat from the chicken; then place the chicken breasts in the bottom of a slow cooker
2. Add the minced garlic and sprinkle with the seasonings
3. Pour in the broth and cover your slow cooker with a lid
4. Cook on High for about 2 to 2 and ½ hours
5. When the time is up, turn off your slow cooker
6. Transfer the chicken breasts into a large bowl; then shred the chicken with two forks

7. Mix the chicken with the rest of ingredients for the different flavoured salads
8. Enjoy the chicken salads on a bed of lettuce greens!

Nutrition Information

Calories: 138.9, Fat: 4.9g, Carbohydrates: 4 g, Protein: 13g, Dietary Fiber 1.7g

Recipe 67: Chicken Cranberry Salad

(Prep time: 5 Mins|Cook Time: 4 Hours| Servings: 4)

Ingredients

- 2 Pounds of skinless and boneless chicken breast
- 1 Pinch of salt and 1 pinch of pepper
- 1 Tablespoon of Tarragon dried
- 1 Cup of diced celery
- 1 Cup of Slivered almonds
- 1 Cup of Cranberries

Instructions

1. Spray your slow cooker with cooking spray
2. Season the chicken breast with 1 pinch of salt and 1 pinch of pepper; then place it into the bottom of your slow cooker
3. Sprinkle the tarragon over the chicken
4. Pour 1 cups of water over the chicken

5. Cover your slow cooker with a lid and cook on High for about 3 to 4 hours or for about 6 to 8 hours on Low
6. Open the slow cooker and shred the chicken with a fork
7. Transfer the chicken to a serving dish and add the almonds and the cranberries to it
8. Serve the chicken into lettuce cups and enjoy!

Nutrition Information

Calories: 277, Fat: 14g, Carbohydrates: 7 g, Protein: 13g, Dietary Fiber 2g

Recipe 68: Shrimp Salad

(Prep time: 5 Mins|Cook Time: 1 Hour| Servings: 3)

Ingredients

- ½ Pound of small peeled and deveined with the tail-off shrimps
- 1 Tablespoon of olive oil
- 1 Teaspoon of jarred minced garlic
- 8 Oz of heart of romaine lettuce leaves
- ½ Cup of halved grape tomatoes
- 1 Small sliced avocado
- 4 tablespoons of Homemade Zesty

Instructions

1. Preheat your slow cooker to Low; then add the olive oil
2. Add the shrimp and pour in 1 tablespoon of water
3. Add the garlic and cover the slow cooker with a lid and cook on High for about 2 Hours on Low
4. When the time is up; turn off your slow cooker

5. Set the shrimp aside to cool
6. Chop the romaine and divide it between two large bowls
7. Top each of the shrimp
8. Serve and enjoy your salads with the dressing!

Nutrition Information

Calories: 237, Fat: 24g, Carbohydrates: 5g, Protein: 22g, Dietary Fiber 0.9g

Recipe 69: Pork salad

(Prep time: 6 Mins|Cook Time: 6 to 8 Hours| Servings: 4)

Ingredients

- 2 Pounds of boneless pork loin roast
- 1 and ½ cups of apple cider or juice
- 1 Can of 4 ounces of drained chopped green chillies
- 3 Minced garlic cloves
- 1 and ½ teaspoons of salt
- 1 and ½ teaspoons of hot pepper sauce
- 1 Teaspoon of chilli powder
- 1 Teaspoon of pepper
- ½ Teaspoon of ground cumin
- ½ Teaspoon of dried oregano
- 12 Cups of torn mixed salad greens
- 2 Medium, chopped tomatoes
- 1 Small chopped red onion

Instructions

1. Place the pork in a 6-qt. slow cooker

2. In a medium bowl, mix the cider with the green chillies, the garlic, the salt, the pepper sauce, the chilli powder, the pepper, the cumin and the oregano
3. Pour the mixture over the pork and cover your slow cooker with a lid
4. Cook on Low for about 6 to 8 hours on Low
5. Remove the pork from the slow cooker and discard the cooking juices and discard the pork
6. Shred the pork with two forks; then arrange the salad green in a serving plate with the salad dressing
7. Top the green with the shredded steak
8. Season with 1 pinch of salt and drizzle a little bit of olive oil
9. Serve and enjoy your salad!

Nutrition Information

Calories: 233, Fat: 8g, Carbohydrates: 11g, Protein: 28g, Dietary Fiber 3g

Recipe 70: Liver salad with hazelnuts

(Prep time: 7 Mins|Cook Time: 2Hours| Servings: 4)

Ingredients

For the salad
- 1Cup of blanched hazelnuts
- 2 Tablespoons of olive oil
- 1 Pound of chopped chicken livers
- 1 and ½ cups of chicken broth
- The juice of ½ a lemon
- 1Cup of sherry vinegar

For the sauce:
- 2 Minced garlic cloves
- Chopped flat-leaf parsley

- 3 Tablespoons of blanched hazelnuts
- 2 tsp of hot smoked paprika
- 4 Tablespoons of olive oil

Instructions

1. Preheat your slow cooker to Low and pour tablespoon of olive oil in it
2. Place the chicken liver in the bottom of your slow cooker and pour the broth into it
3. Cover your slow cooker with a lid and cook on High for about 2 hours
4. Pour the ingredients for the sauce in a food processor and whisk until your ingredients are very well mixed
5. Put the hazelnuts over a baking sheet and roast for about 5 minutes in an oven
6. Turn off your slow cooker and transfer the liver to a large bowl
7. Assemble the salad by adding the sherry to the liver bowl; the lemon juice and 1 pinch of salt
8. Dress the salad with the leaves with a small quantity of sherry vinegar.
9. Spoon the livers and the salad to a serving plate sprinkle with toasted hazel nuts
10. Serve and enjoy your salad!

Nutrition Information

Calories: 298, Fat: 11g, Carbohydrates: 6g, Protein: 26g, Dietary Fiber 2.7g

Whole30 Slow Cooker dessert Recipes

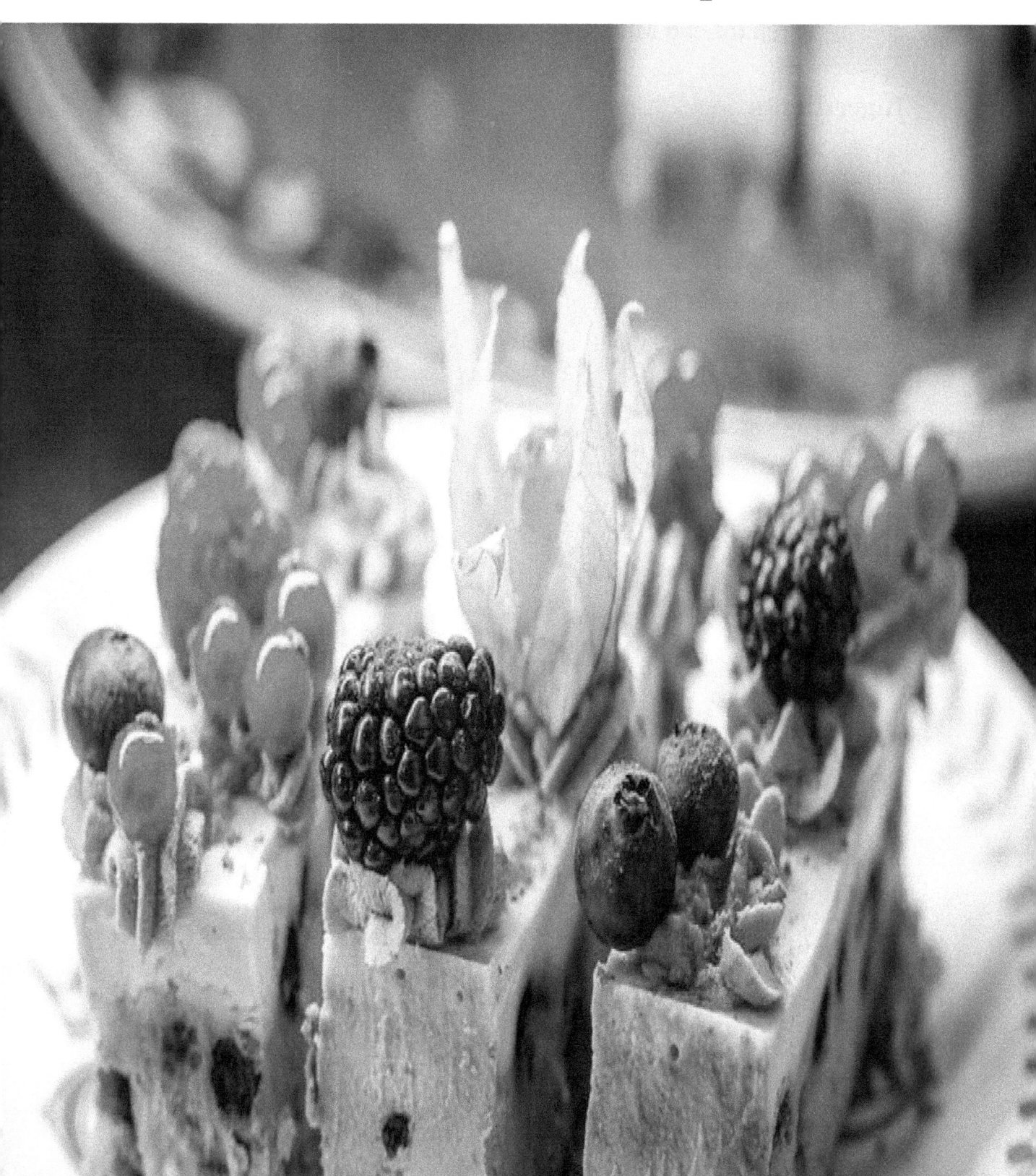

Recipe 71: Apple and cranberry sauce

(Prep time: 6 Mins|Cook Time: 5 Hours| Servings: 3-4)

Ingredients

- 14 Cored, peeled and sliced apples
- 1 Cup of fresh cranberries
- ½ Teaspoon of grated ginger
- 1 Tablespoon of lemon juice
- 1 Teaspoon of pure vanilla extract
- ½ Teaspoon of cinnamon
- 1 Pinch of salt
- ¼ Cup of filtered water

Instructions

1. Place all the ingredients in your slow cooker.
2. Cover your slow cooker with a lid and cook for about 4 to 5 hours on Low
3. Turn off your slow cooker.
4. Break up the apples with a spoon or fork
5. Stir your ingredients very well.
6. Serve and enjoy your dessert!

Nutrition Information

Calories: 100, Fat: 3g, Carbohydrates: 12g, Protein: 3g, Dietary Fiber 2g

Recipe 72: Chocolate fondue

(Prep time: 5 Mins|Cook Time: 1 Hour| Servings: 2)

Ingredients

- 18 Oz of semisweet chopped chocolate
- 1 Oz of unsweetened chopped chocolate
- 6 Oz of chopped 75% dark chocolate
- 1Can of 13 oz of almond milk
- 1 Teaspoon of vanilla
- Fruit cookies

Instructions

1. Combine the chocolates with the almond milk into a 3 quart slow cooker
2. Cover your slow cooker with a lid and cook on Low for about 1 hours
3. When the time is up; turn off your slow cooker; stir very well
4. Add the vanilla and stir
5. Serve and enjoy your dessert!

Nutrition Information

Calories: 164.1, Fat: 6.6g, Carbohydrates: 10.3g, Protein: 2.6g, Dietary Fiber 3.1g

Recipe 73: Sugar-free chocolate fudges

(Prep time: 7 Mins|Cook Time: 4 Hours| Servings: 7)

Ingredients

- 2 and ½ cups of chocolate chips
- ½ Cup of coconut milk
- 1/8 Teaspoon of sea salt
- 1 Teaspoon of vanilla extract

Instructions

1. Grease your slow cooker with coconut oil
2. Pour the coconut milk in a bowl and stir it very well
3. Pour 1 cup of coconut milk in the bottom of your slow cooker and add the remaining ingredients except for the vanilla extract
4. Cover your slow cooker with a lid and cook on High for about 2 hours
5. Add the vanilla; then stir and whisk very well
6. Leave the mixture uncovered for about 3 to 4 hours
7. Stir and grease a 1 container with a little quantity of coconut oil
8. Serve and enjoy your dessert!

Nutrition Information

Calories: 160, Fat: 10g, Carbohydrates: 11g, Protein: 3g, Dietary Fiber 1g

Recipe 74: Stuffed apples

(Prep time: 5 Mins|Cook Time: 1 and ½ Hours| Servings: 5)

Ingredients
- 5 Medium apples with the core hollowed out
- 5 Medium dried figs
- 1 Cup of sugar free date paste
- 1 Teaspoon of chopped crystallized dried ginger
- ¼ Cup of chopped pecans
- ¼ Teaspoon of salt
- ¼ Teaspoon of nutmeg
- ½ Teaspoon of cinnamon
- 1 Teaspoon of lemon zest
- ½ Teaspoon of orange zest
- 1 Tablespoon of fresh lemon juice
- 1 Tablespoon of coconut oil

For the water bath:
- ½ Cup of water
- ½ Teaspoon of cinnamon

Instructions
1. Combine the stuffing ingredients all together
2. Remove the inner centre of each off the apples
3. Stuff the apples with the stuffing; then squeeze the lemon over the top of the apples
4. Pour the water in your slow cooker
5. Place the apples in your slow cooker and cover with the lid
6. Cook on High for about 1 and ½ hours
7. When the time is up, turn off your slow cooker
8. Serve and enjoy your dessert!

Nutrition Information
Calories: 172, Fat: 8.8g, Carbohydrates: 10.9g, Protein: 2.5g, Dietary Fiber 3.2g

Recipe 75: Chocolate clusters

(Prep time: 10 Mins|Cook Time: 2 and ½ Hours| Servings: 3)

Ingredients

- 16 Ounces of salted dry roasted peanuts
- 16 Ounces of unsalted dry roasted peanuts
- 1 Package of dairy-free chocolate chips
- 11 Ounces of white baking chips
- 2 Packages of 75% cacao bittersweet chocolate baking chips

Instructions

1. Combine the peanuts in your slow cooker
2. Add the remaining ingredients and stir
3. Cover your slow cooker with a lid and cook on Low for about 2 and ½ hours on Low
4. When the time is up; turn off your slow cooker and drop the mixture by tablespoons over a waxed paper
5. Place the chocolate clusters in an airtight container
6. Serve and enjoy your chocolate clusters!

Nutrition Information

Calories: 205, Fat: 14g, Carbohydrates: 12g, Protein: 5g, Dietary Fiber 2g

Recipe 76: Slow cooked peaches

(Prep time: 5 Mins|Cook Time: 2 Hours| Servings: 2)

Ingredients
- 3 to 4 peaches
- 1 Teaspoon of coconut oil
- 1 Pinch of cinnamon

Instructions

1. Preheat your slow cooker to Low and spray it with cooking spray
2. Slice the peaches into half and remove the stone
3. Line the slow cooker with cooking spray; then arrange the peaches over it.
4. Pour 1 teaspoon of coconut oil in each of the peach half
5. Cover your slow cooker with the lid
6. Cook on High for about 2 hours on High
7. When the time is up; turn off your slow cooker
8. Serve and enjoy your dessert!

Nutrition Information
Calories: 158.2, Fat: 4g, Carbohydrates: 11g, Protein: 3g, Dietary Fiber 2.1g

Recipe 77: Slow cooked pears with pomegranate

(Prep time: 10 Mins|Cook Time: 4 Hours| Servings: 3)

Ingredients

- 8 to 9 Forelle pears
- 2 Cups of water
- 1 Cinnamon stick
- The rind of an orange
- 1 Cup of water
- 1 Inch of sliced and peeled piece of ginger
- For the garnish:
- 1 Cup of pomegranate arils
- ½ Cup of pistachios
- Orange twists

Instructions

1. Peel the pears and core it; then transfer your ingredients to a slow cooker
2. Add the cinnamon stick, the orange, the ginger and the vanilla. Then cover the slow cooker with a lid and cook on Low for about 3 to 4 hours
3. When the time is up; turn off your slow cooker
4. Serve and enjoy your dessert!

Nutrition Information

Calories: 103.8, Fat: 1.2g, Carbohydrates: 11g, Protein: 2g, Dietary Fiber 2.2g

Recipe 78: Apple sweet potato mash

(Prep time: 10 Mins|Cook Time: 8 Hours| Servings: 3)

Ingredients

- 5 Peeled and chopped apples
- 3 Peeled and chopped sweet potatoes
- ¼ Cup of cinnamon
- 1 Tablespoon of ground ginger
- 1 Tablespoon of pure chocolate powder
- 1 Tablespoon of nutmeg
- ½ Teaspoon of ground cloves

Instructions

1. Place all your ingredients into the bottom of your slow cooker and cover with a lid
2. Cook on Low for about 8 hours
3. When the time is up; turn off your slow cooker
4. Blend your ingredients with an immersion blender and blend your ingredients into a smooth mixture
5. Serve and enjoy your apple sweet potato mash!

Nutrition Information

Calories: 143.7, Fat: 1g, Carbohydrates: 13g, Protein: 2.8g, Dietary Fiber 2.5g

Recipe 79: Slow cooked apple dessert

(Prep time: 4 Mins|Cook Time: 3 Hours| Servings: 4)

Ingredients

- 5 Cups of sliced peeled Granny Smith apples
- 5 Cups of sliced peeled Braeburn apples
- ¼ Cup of almond butter
- 2 Tablespoons of fresh lemon juice
- 2 Teaspoons of ground cinnamon
- ¼ Cup of apple cider

Instructions

1. Spray a 5 to 6 quart slow cooker with cooking spray
2. Combine the apples, the lemon juice; then sprinkle with the cinnamon and toss very well
3. Pour the cider over the apples.
4. Cover your slow cooker with the lid and cook on Low for about 3 hours
5. When the time is up; turn off your slow cooker
6. Serve and enjoy your dessert!

Nutrition Information
Calories: 214, Fat: 4g, Carbohydrates: 12g, Protein: 2g, Dietary Fiber 3g

Recipe 80: Almond granola

(Prep time: 5 Mins|Cook Time: 2 Hours| Servings: 3)

Ingredients

- 1/3 Cup of coconut oil
- 1 Teaspoon of vanilla extract
- 2 Cups of raw almonds, pecans, walnuts and hazelnuts
- 1 Cup of raw sunflower seeds
- 1 Cup of pumpkin seeds
- 1 Cup of unsweetened shredded coconut
- 1 Teaspoon of ground cinnamon
- 1 Teaspoon of salt

Instructions

1. Turn your slow cooker to Low and add in the coconut oil; then let it melt
2. Once the coconut oil is melted, add the vanilla extract
3. Stir your ingredients very well and make sure everything is very well coated
4. Mix the cinnamon with the salt and sprinkle it on top of the nuts and the seeds
5. Cover your slow cooker with a lid and cook on Low for about 2 hours
6. Pour the slow cooked granola over a baking sheet
7. Store the granola in a container; then serve and enjoy it!

Nutrition Information
Calories: 336, Fat: 25g, Carbohydrates: 8.7g, Protein: 7.9g, Dietary Fiber 2.3g

CONCLUSION

Have you ever wondered if you can you change your life by only changing your dietary habits? And did you know that the food you place on your plate can make you healthier than you used to be? If your answer is yes to all the questions; then the Whole30 diet will prove to you that getting into shape and living a healthy life has never been easier.

Since the year 2009, Dallas Hartwig and Melissa Hartwig's came up with a program that helped a huge mass of people lose weight and live with a healthy body and healthy mind. The Whole30diet has proven that it is one of the rare programs that can help you lose weight without exhausting your body with endless exercises.

And not only this diet can help you become healthy effortlessly, but it can help you acquire the confidence you have always dream of; it can improve the quality of your sleep, the levels of energy; it can also improve your mood and self-esteem. Studies have proven that people who have followed the whoel30 diet for just 30 day have experienced a great change in their life; an important decrease in their weight and some of them have managed to get rid of certain serious medical conditions.

The principle of the Whole30 diet is easier than you can imagine; it targets people lives, whether physical or emotional. This diet program is also designed to help cut out with all the unhealthy eating habits; it can stop food-related stress and can reduce the feeling of hunger. Th Whole30 diet is very special because it removes sugar, sugar alternatives, grains and grain alternatives too from your daily meals.

Thus, the main objective of this book is to help your discover some of the most delicious whole30 diet recipes. With 80 recipes that use only a few and affordable ingredients; this whole30 diet book can also help you with its easy-to follow directions; its nutrition information.

The Whole30 diet has spread everywhere in the world; and what is more interesting is that this book focuses on the use of the innovative cooking appliance slow cooker; which can guarantee you tenderness and healthy recipes. Thus, the idea for the Whole30 slow cooker cookbook came improve the function of your digestive system, the function of your brain and even your respiratory system because the whole30 diet eliminates all allergic ingredients from your food. Your will end up realizing that the Whole30 slow cooker diet makes a perfect program for you. And thanks to this Whole30 diet cookbook, you will be able to use the innovative slow cooker cookbook to come up with some of the healthiest and most succulent recipes that you will love.

Thank you for Reading This Book entitled

"The Whole30 Slow Cooker Cookbook

100 Easy and Delicious Recipes For Rapid Weight Loss. Lose Up to 20 Pounds In 21 Days
"

I have shared with you all my knowledge about and strengthened it with my humble dietary experience, some of my favourite recipes, what to eat, what not to eat and everything you need to know about the whole30 diet. I hope, from the bottom of my heart, that you have enjoyed this cookbook and I hope that I have given you enough ideas about this diet. I also wish that the whole30 program does you as good as it did for me and for my friends and family. Feel free to share with us your precious experience with the whole30 diet. If you have any ideas or tips you want to share with me, I would love that. Just keep in mind that Whole30 diet can be hard at first, but you can get used to it in no time. I feel strong with the whole30 diet; I feel healthier emotionally, mentally and physically. I wish you the best of luck with this diet!

www.ingramcontent.com/pod-product-compliance
Lightning Source LLC
Chambersburg PA
CBHW081159020426
42333CB00020B/2555